HANDS-ON YOGA ASSISTS

A Teacher's Guide to The Rubber Band Method®

Kiara Armstrong
ERYT500, CMT, YACEP

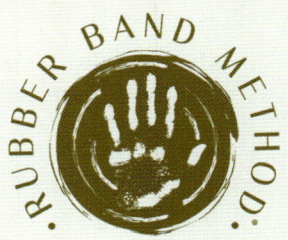

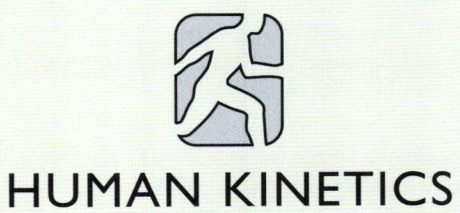

HUMAN KINETICS

Library of Congress Cataloging-in-Publication Data

Names: Armstrong, Kiara, 1982- author
Title: Hands-on yoga assists : a teacher's guide to the rubber band
  method / Kiara Armstrong.
Description: Champaign, IL : Human Kinetics, Inc, [2026] | Includes
  bibliographical references.
Identifiers: LCCN 2024060523 (print) | LCCN 2024060524 (ebook) | ISBN
  9781718238299 paperback | ISBN 9781718238305 epub | ISBN 9781718238312
  pdf
Subjects: LCSH: Yoga | Yoga--Study and teaching | BISAC: HEALTH & FITNESS /
  Yoga | SPORTS & RECREATION / Training
Classification: LCC RA781.67 .A777 2026 (print) | LCC RA781.67 (ebook) |
  DDC 613.7/046076--dc23/eng/20250415
LC record available at https://lccn.loc.gov/2024060523
LC ebook record available at https://lccn.loc.gov/2024060524

ISBN: 978-1-7182-3829-9 (print)

The practices, techniques, and suggestions contained in this book are intended for educational purposes only. While every effort has been made to ensure the accuracy and safety of the content, the author and publisher are not responsible for any injury, discomfort, or adverse effect that may result from your participation in the physical activities described herein. You are solely responsible for your own health, safety, and wellbeing. Always listen to your body and consult with a qualified healthcare provider before beginning any new physical practice, especially if you are pregnant, injured, or have a medical condition. The exercises and assists outlined in this book should be approached with care, awareness, and appropriate professional training. By engaging with this material, you voluntarily assume full responsibility for any risk or injury that may occur and agree to release and discharge the author and publisher from any and all claims or causes of action, known or unknown, arising from the use of this book.

The web addresses cited in this text were current as of December 2024, unless otherwise noted.

Senior Acquisitions Editor: Michelle Earle; **Managing Editor:** Kevin Matz; **Copyeditor:** Kirsten Balayti; **Permissions Manager:** Laurel Mitchell; **Senior Graphic Designer:** Nancy Rasmus; **Layout:** MPS Limited; **Cover Designer:** Keri Evans; **Cover Design Specialist:** Susan Rothermel Allen; **Photographs (cover and interior):** Kiara Armstrong; **Photo Production Manager:** Jason Allen; **Senior Art Manager:** Kelly Hendren; **Illustrations:** © Human Kinetics, unless otherwise noted; **Printer:** Versa Press;

Printed in the United States of America   10   9   8   7   6   5   4   3   2   1

The paper in this book is certified under a sustainable forestry program.

Human Kinetics	*United States and International*	*Canada*
1607 N. Market Street	Website: **US.HumanKinetics.com**	Website: **Canada.HumanKinetics.com**
Champaign, IL 61820	Email: info@hkusa.com	Email: info@hkcanada.com
USA	Phone: 1-800-747-4457	

Human Kinetics' authorized representative for product safety in the EU is Mare Nostrum Group B.V., Mauritskade 21D, 1091 GC Amsterdam, The Netherlands.
Email: gpsr@mare-nostrum.co.uk

E9946

HANDS-ON YOGA ASSISTS

A Teacher's Guide to The Rubber Band Method®

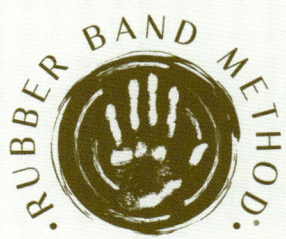

CONTENTS

PART II
Techniques

INTRODUCTION

Before we dive into this instructional manual, I'd like to take you somewhere. Imagine you've stepped onto your yoga mat in a full classroom brimming with yogis and a sense of community. The instructor introduces the vinyasa class, the anatomical focus, and the theme they will thread throughout the practice. The instructor asks you to begin by coming into extended child's pose, with your arms reaching long toward the top of your mat.

The instructor starts to center the room by cuing the breath and inviting you to close your eyes. After a few moments, they say, "In my classes, I like to offer hands-on assists. These are totally optional; I only offer them to provide a little more stretch or grounding to a pose that is already aligned. If you prefer *not* to receive hands-on assists, please give me a thumbs-up with either one or both of your hands. Thank you." You choose to accept the invitation.

As the class proceeds, the instructor fluidly makes their way around the room, assisting students who have opted in. After your third sun salutation, they step into your space and offer a downward dog front press. Your shoulders are just warming up, and the weightless lift of your hips up and back provides a welcome stretch along the sides of your arms and torso. As the instructor finishes the assist, they gently release your body weight and mindfully step out of your space.

The class starts picking up, and the sequence feels a bit too challenging, so you drop to your knees and find child's pose for a few restorative breaths. Moments later, you feel the instructor anchor your sacrum and elongate your spine with a child's pose spinal lengthening. The assist feels reassuring and supportive.

The class begins to wind down, and floor work begins. You feel your ujjayi breath begin to slow and deepen as your body cools. The instructor has guided the class into corpse pose. You are settling a bolster under your knees and a pillow over your eyes when you hear the instructor say, "While you are in corpse pose, I will be offering an assist using lavender essential oil. If you'd prefer *not* to receive this assist, place a hand on your belly for a moment. Thank you." You welcome the assist.

Moments later, your senses are filled with the relaxing aroma of lavender as you hear the instructor softly rubbing their hands together overhead. Their fingers lengthen the back of your neck and palpate the base of your skull, sending waves of relaxation through your entire body with corpse-pose neck traction.

With the soft sound of chimes, you realize the 10-minute savasana has already come to an end. The instructor draws you from your supine position and ends the class by saying, "Namaste." You notice a stillness in your body and a calmness in your mind—the kind of bliss that yoga uniquely creates. You leave feeling fully nourished and intending to return for more. This is an instructor you plan to practice with again and again.

I like to think that I just took you to one of my vinyasa classes, but the class I just described could be any one that offers Rubber Band Method® assists. Over the years, I found that my classes would usually fill up, and I'd often wait-list many students because of the lack of space in the room. As much as I might have wanted to believe that this was due to my sequencing, theming, fun playlists, or anything else concerning my teaching, I always knew it was because of the Rubber Band Method® (RBM) assists I offered in all my classes.

Students simply love receiving energetically and anatomically safe hands-on yoga assists. In addition to resulting in wait-listed classes, RBM assists helped me build a steady clientele of private clients. I was able to offer a unique, one-on-one experience my clients couldn't get in a crowded studio classroom. For years, I saw clients in their homes, offering 60-minute sessions that blended RBM assists with restorative yoga, yin, pranayama, and meditation.

The benefits to a teacher from incorporating RBM assists into their offerings abound. Not only have I experienced this for myself, but I have consistently witnessed an overall increase in student following for the teachers I've trained too. When you offer hands-on yoga assists that are energetically and anatomically safe, your students can feel it. By *safe*, I mean assists that are given only with consent, have a function in the asana practice, and are provided from a steady position by an instructor who knows the anatomy they're touching and the tissues they're affecting.

This book offers an introduction to the Rubber Band Method® and is appropriate for any yoga instructor who wants to conduct safe hands-on assists; it can also supplement both 200-hour and 300-hour yoga teacher training (YTT) programs that aim to train hands-on instructors from the start or deepen existing skills. In this book, you will find everything you need to know to help keep yourself and your students safe when providing foundational assists in yoga classes. I call these assists *foundational* because they are all a teacher will need. The assists in this volume can be used during active or passive parts of the practice, in a packed room or individually. There are more assists that one can and may want to learn in the *Intermediate Use* and *Advanced Applications* books, but the assists in this volume are enough to provide a comprehensive class with assists throughout. It's important to start by learning the assists taught in this volume before considering the more advanced assists in subsequent volumes.

This first volume on the Rubber Band Method® aims to build an instructor's knowledge base so that they can provide safe and helpful touch in the classroom. The concepts covered in this manual include the importance of asking permission and how to do so, the differences between assists and adjustments, the benefits of touch for human health and the asana practice, how to determine which assists to offer to which students, how anatomy and safety inform where and how we touch our students, and why assisting from an unsupported stance is dangerous and uncomfortable for both the teacher and the student. The goal is to help yoga instructors learn how to listen with their hands and read the language of the body's tissues so that every assist can be physically safe for students.

When discussing the use of touch in the classroom, the subject of trauma must be addressed as well. Whether a yoga instructor knows it or not, there are likely students in their classroom who have experienced trauma, and touch can have a significant impact on these students. RBM is not a trauma-informed yoga training; rather, it aims to alert instructors to the issues involved with using touch with individuals who have experienced trauma so that they know how and when to use RBM assists and can do so with confidence and sensitivity. For RBM to be fundamentally safe and helpful for students, instructors must consider both physical and mental or emotional injuries, such as trauma, and make modifications as necessary. I've had complex posttraumatic stress disorder (PTSD) for the better part of my life. Some of my experiences are shared in this book to help teach others about trauma, draw attention to how prevalent trauma can be among students in public classes, and emphasize the benefits touch can have in healing from trauma. Chapter 5, Respectful Assists, shows how RBM can be an effective tool for trauma-informed yoga instructors to add safe touch to their classes.

My hope is that this volume sparks your desire to provide Rubber Band Method® assists to all your students who welcome touch. Not only do I wish you confidence in providing these assists, but I hope that you will come to understand how important touch can be in the yoga classroom and how much benefit assists can add to the asana practice. Yoga is a space for healing, expanding, and training our minds. We do all of this through the doorway of the body. One way we can help our students through that doorway is by providing energetically and anatomically safe touch based on the approach of the Rubber Band Method®.

Rubber Band Method®
Origin, Mission, and Vision

Origin

I created Rubber Band Method® to help others unlock their innate capacity for self-healing. The method emerged from my personal journey navigating the compounded trauma of a long-standing misdiagnosis of complex post-traumatic stress disorder (PTSD). During this painful time, traditional medical treatments repeatedly failed, ultimately prompting me to seek alternative, body-centered healing practices.

For nearly a decade, I lived with severe symptoms and side effects from treatments for a condition I didn't actually have. The compounded trauma from increasingly aggressive medications and dosages eventually culminated in a critical health crisis. A doctor recognized that my intense stress and emotional turmoil likely played a significant role in my declining health and encouraged me to explore holistic ways to support my mental and emotional well-being.

Taking this advice to heart, I immersed myself in practices designed to restore inner calm and emotional resilience, including yoga, meditation, breathwork, and healing-oriented touch. During this period, safe and supportive touch became particularly meaningful, providing a sense of safety, comfort, and grounding at a deeply destabilized time. The experience of receiving such touch significantly improved my emotional well-being and supported my recovery from the acute health crisis within months.

Though I was already familiar with the power of therapeutic touch—having grown up with a massage therapist parent—experiencing safe touch during such a vulnerable healing period amplified my understanding of its profound potential. This realization inspired me to bring safe, purposeful touch into the yoga classroom—creating an environment where students could experience comfort, connection, and a deeper sense of well-being.

Drawing from my own healing, over a decade of teaching yoga while implementing and refining consent-driven, anatomically informed assists, feedback from students, and deep anatomical study as a massage therapist and dissection student, I developed the Rubber Band Method®. Designed specifically for yoga instructors, the method offers a new standard for touch in yoga classrooms.

This journey became the foundation for what is now Rubber Band Method®—a system rooted in teacher and student safety, agency, and the belief that touch, when informed and purposeful, can be profoundly healing.

Mission

Rubber Band Method® sets the standard for anatomically and energetically safe touch in yoga. We offer instructors a structured, accessible system for providing safe, individualized assists and adjustments—grounded in anatomy, sustainable body mechanics, purpose, and tissue reading. Our framework prioritizes both student safety and teacher longevity, empowering classroom environments rooted in personal agency, consent, and trauma sensitivity.

Vision

Rubber Band Method® envisions a world where energetically and anatomically safe touch is integral to the yoga practice. We cultivate a global community of RBM-trained yoga teachers who thrive in their profession—supported by a robust and loyal following of students who seek out and deeply value the benefits of the safe, purposeful touch they incorporate into their teaching. We see consent-based, purposeful touch as a cornerstone of yoga education—enriching the experience of both teachers and students for generations to come.

*While RBM is informed by trauma sensitivity, it is not a clinical intervention or trauma treatment.

HOW TO USE THIS BOOK

Part I of the book—chapters 1 through 6—presents the Rubber Band Method®. Please read this portion first. It's aimed at training you on how to provide safe and helpful touch to your students. These chapters outline aspects of practice that contribute to a safe classroom environment. They also note the science behind this approach to hands-on assisting and the subsequent benefits. Chapters 1 through 6 are best read in order, but once you've mastered these topics, you can bounce around part II of the book (chapters 7-11) to reference how to offer a specific assist or refine a certain stance.

Chapters 7 through 11 don't need to be read in order, nor were their topics intended to be learned in a specific order. The assists are presented by pose name, separated by the anatomical focus of the assist, and listed in alphabetical order. The assists are not listed from easiest to most challenging. Instead, I invite you to jump to the assist you want to bring into your classroom. Are you a vinyasa teacher and teach a lot of downward-facing dog? Go to the Downward Dog: Front Press section in chapter 10 for an overview of the assist. You will find that warrior I is one of the stances instructors use to offer this assist. Refine that stance by reading about it in detail in chapter 7. Or perhaps you are a mellow flow instructor, and you frequently teach child's pose in your class. In this case, you can find overviews of the assists for child's pose in chapters 9 and 10 and details on the applicable stances in chapter 7.

This volume isn't intended to be read from cover to cover. It would be extremely difficult to learn and remember all 15 assists in one cover-to-cover reading. Instead, learn the methodology in chapters 1 through 6, and then choose to learn one assist and its stance at a time. As you grow more and more comfortable, learn an additional assist. You can find more details in the Suggestions for Learning section in chapter 6.

PART

I

METHODOLOGY

1

THE SCIENCE OF
SAFE TOUCH

Thankfully, over recent years, science has turned its eye toward body-centric methods for maintaining health and supporting healing. Although it's still common for people to look outside themselves for the answers to health and well-being, many researchers have started to study what wisdom our evolutionarily ancient bodies can provide about homeostasis and healing from the inside out.

We receive myriad messages from our bodies throughout the day and even into the night with our sleep. These messages communicate the state of our well-being and whether something we're experiencing has a positive, negative, or neutral effect. These messages can be simple, subtle, or painfully (literally) obvious. For the most part, though, the signals the body sends are very subtle, and to notice them requires a certain degree of body awareness. We'll delve into body awareness and how to improve it in the next chapter, but for now, understand that all the messages sent from the body to the mind and the mind to the body are delivered and sensed via the nervous system.

The nervous system plays possibly the most important role in our well-being or *dis*-ease because it's what connects the brain and mind with the body and makes them essentially inseparable. The nervous system is how we have come to understand that our thoughts and emotions affect our physical health and that our physical state can affect our mental state. Because of this inextricable connection between mind and body via the nervous system, the nervous system has become the number one way we can "hack" our biology, or disrupt patterns that might be causing dis-ease or disease and change them toward patterns of ease and healing.

Scientific research now demonstrates that body-centric practices like exercise, yoga, breath work, and touch play a significant role in health and well-being because we can use the body to influence the mind. This matters because the mind is a powerful yet elusive thing that can feel difficult to regulate—most yogis know how true this is! However, we can literally touch the body, and because of its very tangible nature, it can feel more accessible than the mind. When we positively affect the body, it benefits the mind, and vice versa. This creates a circular process: tapping into the body impacts the mind, which in turn affects the body—back and forth it goes. This circular exchange, whether positive or negative, occurs through the nervous system. When we get to know the nervous system, we begin to understand why body-centric techniques have such a widespread impact on the organism, or what you think of as you and your body.

Keeping this in mind, let's look at some scientific research on the positive effects of touch as a body-centric healing aid. Then, we'll dive into the nitty-gritty as to why we see these positive effects of touch on human health via the nervous system.

THE BENEFITS OF SAFE TOUCH

For a long time, the research on the benefits of touch for human health largely focused on babies. However, a recent meta-analysis[1] of many research studies on touch proved that touch is powerfully beneficial for adults too. In fact, the research is so convincing that touch is beneficial to our health that one can deduce that it's vital to health and well-being.

The meta-analysis revealed that touch is especially effective for easing pain and reducing anxiety and depression in adults and children. Touch even has the power to help buffer against or reduce future stress and anxiety. The research revealed that it doesn't matter who is providing touch, which means that touch can be beneficial regardless of whether it comes from a trained massage therapist, a best friend, or a yoga instructor providing Rubber Band Method® (RBM) assists. However, consent is paramount when considering the benefits of touch for human health; the touch must be consensual. Touch that isn't consensual can be harmful, even traumatic.

The meta-analysis considered various kinds of consensual touch and noted that all forms have a positive impact. The duration of touch, such as a full-body massage versus a brief touch, wasn't key. In fact, the data showed more significant benefit when touch was received more frequently rather than for longer periods of time—think receiving hands-on yoga assists daily in your yoga class versus your once-a-month massage. Research proves, across hundreds of studies, that consensual touch is good for one's health. This research supports the positive impact RBM assists can have on students. The RBM teacher really can amplify the benefits of a student's asana practice.

And why not? We already integrate *pranayama, bandha, dristi,* and *mudra* to help focus the mind and enrich the experience of *asana*—safe, supportive, purposeful touch is simply another tool that achieves the same goals.

TOUCH AND THE NERVOUS SYSTEM

Now that we know that touch is powerfully beneficial to our health, let's consider why. Touch's implications for our overall health are directly linked to stress reduction and tapping into the nervous system. The body is governed by the autonomic nervous system, which comprises the sympathetic branch, which controls stress or active responses, and the parasympathetic branch, which controls rest and passive responses. When your body is in a state of stress, it activates the hypothalamus–pituitary gland–adrenal gland (HPA) response via the sympathetic branch of the autonomic nervous system.

The HPA axis is quick and efficient at flooding the body with the stress molecules cortisol, epinephrine, and norepinephrine. These hormones and neurotransmitters are essential and needed by our bodies for normal organ function. For example, cortisol helps us wake up in the morning and plays an important role in our circadian rhythms, or our wake–sleep cycles. However, the adage "too much of a good thing" applies here. When we're constantly in a state of stress, these molecules will start to damage our organs, cause fatigue, create a racing mind, and even lead to unwanted weight gain. Unfortunately, industrialized Western cultures often promote a mentality of constant activity, as reflected in sayings like "no pain, no gain" and "I'll rest when I die." Constant activity puts us in a perpetual state of stress that the body can't handle indefinitely.

A perpetual state of stress manifests a multitude of disruptions because the body is basically in fight-or-flight mode at all times—that is, preparing itself to respond to perceived threats. A constantly racing mind leads to disrupted sleep or insomnia, which is deleterious for the brain and other organ systems. When the body is perpetually prepared for fight or flight, it chronically activates the musculoskeletal system. With constant activation of the musculoskeletal system, we see symptoms of inexplicable chronic pain, especially lower back pain. Furthermore, disturbed digestion and gastric problems arise (e.g., irritable bowel syndrome [IBS], for which health care providers often prescribe an antidepressant to resolve the gastric issue), focus becomes impaired because of the predominance of beta brainwaves, and some regions of the brain even atrophy.

Treating chronic stress can prove to be difficult for many. So, what options do we have? We can find the answer in the other branch of the autonomic nervous system. The parasympathetic nervous system governs our "chill-out" or shut-off response. It is the inhibitory branch of the autonomic nervous system. Its most valuable player is the vagus nerve, the 10th cranial nerve, which is responsible for our sense of safety and feelings of relaxation, as well as for signaling to the body that it's time to repair itself. When you're constantly "going" or in a perpetual state of stress, your body considers this a stimulated environment where you aren't safe, and processes necessary for digestion, cell repair, and reproduction don't function as well because preparing for impending escape or confrontation is more important to keep you alive. The point is, when you're chronically stressed, your body doesn't feel safe, so it won't allocate resources toward functions that are otherwise not needed in an emergency. Those processes can only function optimally when both your mind and body feel safe.

Cultivating balance between the two branches—the sympathetic and the parasympathetic systems—is essential for health and well-being. Both branches serve a vital purpose; each is equally important. When we're in a state of good health, each branch will do its part in a give-and-take sort of way. For example, the sympathetic branch helps you perform well in your sweaty vinyasa class, but your parasympathetic branch helps you catch your breath, slow your heart rate, and get into that "zen place" in savasana. This is what the respective branches do naturally: They work in tandem to create a kind of back-and-forth equilibrium.

Balancing the Branches of the Nervous System

What's important to remember about the nervous system is that it's adaptable, just like everything else in the body; we can train it in a maladaptive or positively adaptive way. We can train our branches to be balanced, as in the previous example of the vinyasa class, or we can train them to be out of balance, where one of the branches is stronger or more dominant than the other.

Let's explore this concept further with an analogy. We can compare the balance between the two branches of the autonomic nervous system to driving a car. To successfully drive to and arrive at any destination, you need to use both the gas and brake pedals, alternating between the two. In this analogy, the sympathetic branch of the nervous system is the gas; it's your "get-up-and-go" feeling, providing momentum and acceleration. The brake is the parasympathetic branch, which is the opposite of the gas; it slows us down when we're going too fast, gives us a moment of pause, or can bring us to a full stop. This is how the two branches work in our bodies as well: The sympathetic provides the acceleration, and the parasympathetic provides the brakes. The two signal our bodies, back and forth, like the gas and brake pedals signal a car to ensure we arrive safely at our destination. Just like driving requires that you use both pedals, in the body, both branches are always working together; one branch isn't perpetually on and the other perpetually off. However, one branch can become stronger and be recruited more frequently than the other.

The heart is a beautiful example of this balance and one direct means to see how well our two branches are balanced. Every time you inhale, the sympathetic branch activates, and the heart quickens a little. Every time you exhale, the parasympathetic branch activates, and the heart slows a little. The signals sent to your heart by the "gas" (sympathetic branch) and the "brake" (parasympathetic branch) cause this quickening and slowing effect; the time measured between the beats is called *heart-rate variability* (HRV).

High HRV is ideal because it demonstrates how well the two branches are working together. With low HRV, the time between beats is relatively similar, which often indicates a predominance in sympathetic activity. Sympathetic dominance is like pressing the gas pedal to the metal—full acceleration. The parasympathetic branch is trying to hit the brakes, but the gas is fully pressed, and the brake doesn't do much to slow the acceleration. Hence, the time between beats becomes similar because the parasympathetic branch isn't effectively slowing the heart.

Conversely, high HRV means there is variation rather than consistency in the time between beats. When the brake is applied, the heart slows. This is like smooth driving—sometimes we use the gas pedal, sometimes the brake. The back-and-forth between the two branches creates variation from beat to beat, representing a balance between the two branches.

Toning the Nervous System

When you've toned your sympathetic branch to go, go, go, it can be tough to shift out of a stressed state at will. Being in a constant state of stress is like *practicing* being stressed, and your sympathetic branch becomes stronger and more dominant. Such activation is called *tone*, and I like to think of it just like muscle tone. When you target your biceps muscle with exercise or use it frequently, it gets stronger and more toned over time. When you tone or use one of the nervous system branches predominately, it can become more proficient and stronger over time.

The more you recruit a sympathetic response, such as being stressed, the more easily it is recruited, which means it's easier for you to get stressed. Toning of the sympathetic branch via chronic stress usually means the parasympathetic branch isn't getting activated or toned much at all. Without the regular activation of your parasympathetic branch, it loses its tone, and you lose the ability to override a stress response. This is demonstrated in the example of the heart and low HRV. When we aren't regularly using, strengthening, and toning the parasympathetic nervous system, it loses its ability to balance the system, and our bodies miss out on the repair they need.

So, what might this look like in real life? When I had posttraumatic stress disorder (PTSD), I was perpetually in a state of fight or flight and suffered from chronic pain as a result. The predominance of stress in my body manifested in myriad ways (e.g., extremely low HRV), but one pronounced example was my unceasing joint, neck, and back pain. As mentioned earlier, when the nervous system constantly feels like it needs to be ready to run from a perceived threat, the musculoskeletal system becomes chronically activated, and the muscles move into a state of hypertonicity. *Hypertonicity* is when the muscles stay clenched without you always being aware of it. It wasn't until I got my nervous system in balance, lessened my stress, and strengthened my ability to relax that I found relief.

When we regularly activate or engage the parasympathetic nervous system via the vagus nerve, we build its tone. Frequent activation of the vagus nerve is called *vagal toning*. Having strong vagal tone helps bring balance to the nervous system by training the parasympathetic branch to be prepared to mediate the stress response. When we tone the parasympathetic nervous system, symptoms from chronic stress can be alleviated, as demonstrated in my own experience of chronic pain. Moreover, HRV increases, and we start to see the entire body move itself back into a state of homeostasis, or balance. Our systems operate more smoothly as we shift between the "gas pedal" and the "brake."

Toning Through Touch

So, how do we start using our internal brake more often? How do we shift out of being chronically stressed and move into a state of calm relaxation at will? Yoga, with its asana, breathing, meditation, and mantra practices, can help to activate or tone the parasympathetic nervous system, as can listening to music. However, while engaging in these activities, you can still be thinking about your to-do list, replaying that conflict for the thousandth time in your head, or worrying about another stressor. Touch, on the other hand, seems to override the mind and quickly disrupt the stress response. Research has proven that touch can reduce cortisol levels, demonstrating the physiological reduction of stress occurring in the body. This is considered a *bottom-up* regulation method because the body creates a sense of safety and calm rather than the mind.

Touch that feels safe stimulates the vagus nerve, and research shows that the vagus nerve acts as the gatekeeper for repair within the body. Touch—specifically, the feeling of safety when being touched—quickly induces a sense of relaxation, *which is the felt experience of parasympathetic activation*. When you practice relaxation, you are toning the parasympathetic nervous system.

Research has linked relaxation to brainwave states such as theta and delta waves, which occur during meditation and sleep. These brainwaves are important for brain health and keeping regions of the brain from atrophy; thus, the more we cultivate these brainwaves, the better it is for our overall health. When your brain "practices," or uses these waves on a regular basis, the waves can be induced more easily, leading to improved attention, improved sleep, and enhanced relaxation. Being able to relax easily indicates that one's parasympathetic branch is well toned.

Research has also linked touch to an increase in oxytocin. Oxytocin is often called the "bonding molecule," but it's much more than that. Oxytocin increases our sense of trust and improves sociability. It helps to reduce inflammation in the body and lowers the heart rate and stress. Loneliness is becoming a major social epidemic, and oxytocin is an antidote because it makes us feel connected to others. In general, it lifts our spirits and helps us feel connected with and more compassionate toward others.

In addition to resulting in the release of oxytocin, doesn't safe touch simply feel good? Two neurotransmitters linked to "feeling good" are dopamine and serotonin. Dopamine is important for helping us feel fulfilled, rewarded, and contented. I think of dopamine as the felt sense of "*aaaaaahhhhh.*" Serotonin is what many pharmaceutical drugs used to treat psychiatric conditions, such as depression and anxiety, aim to target. This is because serotonin is linked to happiness and improved mood. Our brains and guts create serotonin themselves from the nutrients we provide our bodies, but if we're in a chronic state of stress, serotonin production can be affected, and we start to feel low and depressed.

Receiving safe touch is truly vital to our health and well-being. However, in many cultures, touch is limited. At most, we might get the occasional welcome or goodbye hug, a tap on the shoulder when we say something funny, or an occasional hand-holding. Biologically, this isn't enough. As the mental health crisis and epidemics of loneliness and stress soar, we need more safe touch in the world. We need more safe touch that is easily accessible and frequently experienced. Imagine what our world would look like with less loneliness and stress. Imagine the very real impact RBM assists can have on your students and your community. Years and years of experience have proven to me that students feel the benefits; hence, this is why RBM teachers see their following grow. People want more consensual touch because they can feel the benefits for both their body and mind.

2
CLARIFYING TERMS

ADJUSTMENT VERSUS ASSIST

We create the culture in our classrooms via the words we use, whether those words are in our native tongue or Sanskrit, so an accurate description of how we employ touch in class is necessary. As instructors, we need to give students a clear understanding of the different meanings of the term *touch*—for example, how we might use touch to correct versus how we might use it to add stretch, grounding, or ease.

When I first introduced Rubber Band Method® (RBM) assists to existing teachers, they often said to me, "I prefer to use my words rather than my hands to adjust my students," and I couldn't agree with them more. We should *always* use words when we correct a student. But what about when we aren't correcting a student? What do we call touch that we use to assist stretching, grounding, or ease?

We can't use the word *adjustment* for this kind of touch because *adjustment* literally means "to correct," which is not our aim when adding stretch, grounding, or ease. So, we're right to use the word *adjustment* to refer to the touch we employ to correct our students, but when we use touch in other ways, the word *adjustment* falls short. A better word to describe employing touch to support added stretch, grounding, and ease is *assist* because this kind of touch *assists* the pose rather than *corrects* the pose.

TOUCH AND PROPRIOCEPTION

Touch, in general, via adjustments and assists, has its place in the yoga practice. As the instructor offering touch interventions, it's our job to understand the role adjustments and assists play within the practice and when and how we, as instructors, should offer these techniques in class. The foundational benefit of such an understanding is that we can use it to help the student improve and hone their proprioceptive awareness—that is, the level to which the student is attuned to their body.

Proprioception, which involves sensing and interpreting the body's cues, including postural and positional feedback, as well as knowing where one's body is in space, is a key aspect of body awareness. We might offhandedly assume that everyone is walking around with keen body awareness, but that simply isn't true. Proprioceptive awareness varies widely from person to person. In fact, some students are disembodied and feel little to no connection to their bodies at all (more on this in chapter 5).

Yoga strengthens proprioceptive awareness significantly because it challenges the body's physical strength, flexibility, and balance. All three of these demands on the body provide kinesthetic feedback, or messages from one's body. Being able to interpret kinesthetic feedback is body awareness. Put more simply, we get a lot of different kinds of signals from our bodies from the various ways in which yoga challenges us. Over time, as we become more accustomed to receiving these cues in practice, we learn to better hear the messages from our bodies, thus improving our body awareness, or proprioception.

When we use an adjustment to correct a student's alignment, they learn to *feel* what safe alignment is in that pose. This felt sense of alignment is proprioception. When we assist them with added stretch, grounding, or ease in poses, they grasp a greater felt sense of each; the proprioceptive messages of stretch, grounding, or ease become more pronounced. We may take our proprioceptive awareness for granted as seasoned yogis and instructors, barely noticing our body awareness as a skill. However, for many novice and even intermediate yoga students, attuned proprioceptive awareness is a skill they are still honing. For students with trauma, it's a skill that's vital for healing and embodiment.

Body awareness is profoundly important in both obvious and subtle ways, from sensing pain or danger to interpreting a gut feeling (termed *interoception*) and even being able to tune in to early signs of illness or disease. It's proprioception that precipitates presence and the yoga bliss that we, as teachers of the practice, have come to know and love!

Awareness Is Like a Nesting Doll

Body awareness starts with proprioception, or being able to sense your body in space and feel its physical cues. Once you've honed your proprioception, you can acquire a subtler form of body awareness, termed *interoception*. Interoception involves the ability to sense your pulse, heartbeat, and breath. Interoception also involves the ability to sense gut feelings. Both proprioception and interoception, collectively termed *body awareness*, help you cultivate self-awareness. I like to think of self-awareness as *egoception*, which is our ability to observe thoughts and emotions and their effect within and on the body.

Both adjustments and assists are based on alignment. We provide an adjustment when we see that the student is *out of alignment.* In contrast, we can provide an assist when we see that the student is *in alignment.* So, adjustments and assists are similar in that they're both based on alignment, but they differ in that we offer one when a student is out of alignment, and we offer the other when a student is in alignment. Because we offer adjustments for safety reasons, they are necessary. In contrast, because assists merely add something extra to a student's already safe practice, they are *totally optional*—a bonus for entraining proprioception and embodiment.

The RBM Definition of Alignment

Alignment is a general framework with which we build a pose, helping to differentiate between asanas (e.g., distinguishing Warrior I from Warrior II) by understanding how to position the body in various ways to embody different poses across multiple planes and ranges of motion. Without alignment, we wouldn't have open-hip or closed-hip poses, twists, or inversions; alignment serves as a foundational guide for constructing each pose.

For the most part, the basic alignment of each pose is designed to ensure joint safety while facilitating stretch, challenging balance, and/or building strength. Alignment is intended as a flexible framework that can be tailored by the practitioner to meet their unique needs rather than as a rigid "cookie cutter" structure. Being "in alignment" prioritizes joint safety and honors the individual's natural range of motion while maintaining the integrity of the intended pose.

In the context of hands-on assisting, alignment ensures the pose provides accessible, stable handholds and demonstrates clear directional lines for the teacher to follow when offering an assist. Being in alignment also indicates the student is in a variation of the pose that is safe, comfortable, and appropriate for an assist to enhance their practice without causing strain or misalignment.

YOGA ADJUSTMENTS

Now that we have a basic understanding of the value of and similarities between adjustments and assists and their role in safe alignment and honing proprioception, let's consider each in greater detail. We'll start with yoga adjustments.

Adjust (ə-jŭst′)

To move or change (something) so as to be in a more effective arrangement or desired condition.

To change so as to be suitable to or conform with something else: synonym: adapt.[1]

As you can see from its definition, *adjustment* is the accurate word to describe a teacher's aim to move or change the alignment of their student. An adjustment usually occurs when the teacher corrects the student for safer alignment. We make a correction or adjustment with verbal cues, and we might also include touch, such as providing a light tactile cue, demonstrating a variation of the pose, or providing the student with props to help correct their alignment.

Regardless of how the instructor chooses to correct, the instructor should always use verbal cues to make an adjustment. The aim of an adjustment is for the student to learn what the safe alignment should be for their body in each pose. Verbalizing the correction helps to reinforce this learning.

I suggest using verbal cues first to make an adjustment. A student who has refined proprioceptive awareness will likely respond to verbal cues easily and accurately; the student will sense the various parts of their body that are out of safe alignment and will be able to make micro-adjustments to correct it. However, not all students have cultivated an acute sense of proprioceptive awareness, and verbal cues might not be enough for each student to understand how to correct their form. So, in addition to verbal cues, we can also use light tactile cues, demonstrations of variations of the pose, and modifications with props to correct for safe alignment.

When using light tactile cues with verbal cues, the teacher is not moving the students themselves but rather using light touch to help signal where the student can find safe alignment. For example, when the student is in warrior II, lightly placing your hand outside their front knee and stating, "Press your knee toward my hand," can help the student understand how to abduct or press their knee out more to avoid caving the knee in this pose. Conversely, if the teacher were to push the knee into alignment, the student wouldn't feel the action required in their hip to abduct and maintain safe alignment through the knee.

When we adjust students with light tactile cues, they move themselves into safe alignment. When students correct and move themselves, they are honing their proprioceptive awareness and building muscle memory, which will help them find that safe alignment the next time they practice the pose. Put another way, when the teacher forcibly moves the student into safe alignment, the student doesn't cultivate the proprioception to find that safe alignment next time because they didn't do it themselves. Furthermore, when a teacher forcibly moves a student who is in a pose that's already compromised and potentially unsafe, they risk making matters worse, and injury can occur.

Adjustments may require more than light tactile cues because students may need more specific guidance, or a student may not wish to be touched. Another option for adjusting a pose is to demonstrate a modified variation of the pose in front of or beside students to show them how to adjust themselves into safer alignment if they are struggling with the current variation of the pose the class is working on.

An adjustment can also involve giving a student blocks, a blanket, or a strap to help them achieve safety in their alignment. An adjustment aims to move the student into a *more effective arrangement or desired condition*, and that doesn't always mean solely modifying their body; props are sometimes necessary to make the correction. After giving the prop to the student, verbally cue them on how to align their body safely with the help of the prop.

Ask Yourself

The Yoga Sutras tell us that we should always practice asana with steadiness and ease. This is a good intention to have when adjusting your students. When considering an adjustment, I invite you to ask yourself, "How can I guide my student into greater steadiness and ease in this pose?"

As mentioned earlier, forcibly moving a student into a safer alignment is not the appropriate way to use touch to adjust our students.
Let's consider a real-life example and all the reasons why we don't
use forceful touch to correct or adjust our students.

Let's imagine the instructor is teaching revolved triangle. They
notice that one of their students is far out of alignment, with their
hips swiveled (resulting in concern for knee and spine safety), their
front knee bent (resulting in concern for hamstring-attachment tear),
their shoulders rounded (resulting in lower back vulnerability), and
their arms struggling to find the "T" position (resulting in instability
in balance or concern for general strain). In this scenario, the teacher
should not walk over and forcibly move their student into a safer
alignment; doing so would create more risk of injury for the student.
Let's consider some of those risks and pitfalls to adjusting a student
by forcibly moving them into a safer shape.

For example, what if their form is due to a hamstring or shoulder
injury? If the teacher moves them into alignment instead of directing
them with a light tactile cue regarding where they need to go (hips
back, chest forward, etc.), they risk further injuring these already
vulnerable areas. With light tactile guidance, the teacher can feel
where the student's body resists or stops, signaling to the teacher
that the student cannot go farther in that direction. Teachers may
easily miss this feedback when they use a forcible adjustment.

Let's imagine that in this example, the student's hips are swiveled
because their front hamstring group has an old tear injury, and they
feel too tight to align their hips and spine to neutral. They have swiveled their hips toward the front leg to give their front hamstrings
additional slack. With the lightest touch directing the front hip back,
the teacher will feel when the student's body stops and cannot move
farther toward neutral. The teacher will even notice that what is pre-
venting correct alignment is the front leg. Looking at the student's
rounded shoulders and other clues, the teacher will realize that the
student needs blocks to get to a neutral pelvis. The teacher should
bring the blocks to the student and demonstrate the safe form beside
them. If the student still doesn't understand safe form, the teacher
can use light touch and verbal cues to direct the front hip back and
into neutral alignment when the student is using blocks.

As another example, consider a student who isn't injured; they're
just relatively new to the practice and still improving their proprio-

ceptive awareness. If the teacher elects to move the student into safer alignment, the teacher does it for the student, and the student doesn't get the opportunity to learn how to find safe alignment on their own. This is problematic if the teacher hopes for the student to find safe alignment next time. When the student finds the alignment on their own, they are better able to remember and repeat the alignment. This ongoing practice of self-correcting and modifying the poses is how one hones proprioception and is part of what each yogi learns through their practice. A teacher should not take that opportunity away from students.

Additionally, moving the student can get messy, particularly in a shape like revolved triangle. If the teacher forcibly moved the student's feet, hips, shoulders, and so forth, the student would likely fall over and end up feeling less capable than when they started. If you aim to empower your students, give them the ability to find the safe alignment on their own with your gentle guidance.

In all these examples of how to adjust students, the aim is to keep students safe while supporting their learning process to the best of our ability. When we distill what an adjustment is, it's providing a change to the pose to make it safer and more sustainable for the student's unique body while supporting them in learning from the practice.

Yoga Adjustment

A change to a pose to make it safer and more sustainable for the student's unique body while supporting them in learning from the practice

A correction made to a pose using verbal cues to support learning alignment

A change or correction to a pose that may employ light tactile cues, demonstration , or props

YOGA ASSISTS

Now, let's take a deeper look at assists and what we'll be learning to do in this book. Heading back to the dictionary, let's consider the definition:

Assist (ə-sĭst′)

To give help or support to, especially as a subordinate or supplement; aid.

To give aid or support.[2]

Here, the definition shows us an accurate word to describe a teacher's aim to support or supplement their student's asana practice with additional stretch, grounding, or ease. We are applying a touch intervention to aid the practice; it *assists* the pose. In its current state, the student's practice doesn't need correcting or changing, but by adding an assist, the student might experience a greater felt sense of stretch, grounding, or ease from the pose.

Instructors should offer assists with firm but receptive touch that has a clear direction or directional pressure. All assists should mimic the actions of the pose, accentuate the lines of stretch felt within the shape, or follow the alignment lines of the pose to serve an obvious purpose in the student's practice. The goal is not to fix or change a student's shape or make it more advanced. Beyond asking permission to touch, a basic yoga assist doesn't require verbal guidance or cues.

Choosing the right student to assist is crucial. Assists should only be offered to students who are safely aligned, holding the pose comfortably, and without known injuries affected by the assist. It's essential to ensure the student is in a variation of the pose that can be assisted and to avoid assisting students with known injuries in areas that would be affected by the assist. Additionally, the instructor must have enough space around the student to establish a secure stance and access appropriate handholds.

Focus on students whose alignment provides clear lines to follow or accentuate. If a student's variation of the pose or alignment does not clearly support safe and effective assisting, offering an assist could unintentionally introduce instability or risk.

Ask About Injuries or Pain

It's essential for yoga instructors to ask their students about any injuries, surgeries, or pain; it is important to ask about all three because sometimes students are only aware of pain but may not have had a specific injury or surgery. Yoga poses result in significant demands on the tissues and joints, and hands-on yoga assists can increase these demands, which could exacerbate injuries or pain.

After teaching for several years, I know firsthand that many students don't tell their teacher about their injuries; they think it's not important. However, it's necessary to be fully informed as an asana instructor and as an RBM teacher who offers assists because this information is vital to performing assists safely.

You may ask students about injuries in any number of ways. Here are a couple of examples:

- If it's an intimate studio setting and you're checking in your students as they arrive, ask them individually: "How's your body feeling today—anything I should know about? Any significant pain, injuries, or surgeries?"
- If it's a packed studio environment and you aren't checking in your students individually, announce to the class a couple of times as people are setting up their mats: "Welcome, everyone, as you're getting settled, please come say hi and let me know of any pain, injury, or surgeries that you're bringing to your mat today."

In my classes, I have always sequenced and geared the postures toward an anatomical focus and apex pose. I made it a practice to start asking students to let me know if they had any injuries or pain in the specific joints or regions that we would be focusing on that day. For example, I'd ask about the lumbar spine if we were working on camel pose, or I'd ask about the hips if we were working toward mermaid pose. By focusing my classes on specific poses, I could then ask students about specific sites, and this made students more likely to tell me about their conditions because I was specifically asking about the hips, low back, and so forth.

An informed teacher is an impactful teacher who is in the best position to ensure the safety of their students. Keep communication open, and learn about what your students bring to their mats.

An assist is offered with firm pressure that directs the tissues along the action lines of the pose. When the instructor follows the alignment, mimics the actions of the pose, or accentuates the lines of stretch, the purpose of the assist is obvious to the student. The technique *assists* the pose; it creates more of what the student is already feeling in the pose, whether that's more stretch, grounding, or ease.

For example, when attempting locust-pose foot anchor, many students struggle with the competing actions of rooting the tops of all 10 toes down while simultaneously trying to lift the torso into a backbend. When you provide the anchoring assist to the feet, the student experiences how much more they can extend the backbend when they truly ground all 10 toes, offering more ease in their overall effort and more stretch to the entire front of their body.

As mentioned, an assist never aims to make a pose more advanced. When assisting, we always follow or accentuate the lines of the shape. As a result, if someone were watching the assist, it would look like very little has changed because change is not the intention. However, the student experiences greater lengthening, expansion, opening, and grounding. Because of this, sometimes a student will fold deeper, dip back farther, or lengthen longer. When this happens, the student's body has gone there with your support, not because you forced them there.

Practicing Aparigraha in Poses

Who hasn't, at some point, fallen into grasping, or parigraha, for the most advanced or "perfect" pose? In my decades of practice, I've been the student who struggled to attain the most complex variation of poses and forced myself into idealized shapes—to my body's detriment. I was also the student who let teachers push, pull, and force my body toward that advanced bind, backbend, fold, and so forth, and my body experienced many tissue tears as a result. This striving for more advanced poses can be seen everywhere—in one's personal practice, in the classroom, and on social media.

However easy it might be to fall into the practice of grasping, or parigraha, for the most advanced expression of a pose, the Yoga Sutras tell us that to truly practice yoga, we must do it with aparigraha, which is nongrasping. On the yogic path, aparigraha looks like doing the work without having an attachment to the outcome. As presented in the sutras, having detachment from the fruits of one's labor applies to everything in life, including the asana practice.

There's an old saying by Lao Tzu, "When the student is ready, the teacher will appear." With a little rephrasing, I think this applies to one's asana practice as well: "When the body is ready, the pose will appear." If we, as teachers, are attempting to force a student's body into a shape against the clear pulling back or resistance of their tissues, the body is not ready for that pose! Injuries can occur in yoga when the body is forced into shapes that it isn't ready for or that it didn't get into on its own.

Using RBM, we can support the student's body to step into more advanced poses on its own, when it's ready, through simple support rather than by exerting any amount of force.

When you offer an assist, the felt experience of a pose is accentuated. Have you ever noticed how much more deeply your torso and shoulders stretch in downward dog when you get an assist versus when you hold the pose on your own? Or how calming and grounding a chest press can be in reclined bound angle? Have you ever experienced how assists involving the feet in corpse pose quickly draws you out of rumination and back into your body? All assists accentuate the action, intent, or overall experience of the pose. With this in mind, if the student looks like they are at their limit, accentuating the felt sense of the pose isn't necessary and an assist shouldn't be given to that student.

I especially like to use assists to support students who choose to skip challenging portions of vinyasa practice and instead find child's pose. In a way, it's a great act of courage and self-love for a student to break away from the rest and drop to their knees in a passive pose when the class has become too challenging. When I see a student choose child's pose over downward dog, the apex pose, or a challenging krama (wave of poses), I will support them in their choice by giving them a child's pose assist. I know that when I receive an assist in these moments, I feel acknowledged, encouraged, and supported by my teacher. This is yet another example of how an assist can support the student's pose and practice.

So, which students should you offer an assist to? It can be any student in your room who has consented to touch, has no relevant injuries or pain, demonstrates clear and safe alignment, is comfortably holding their pose, and provides clear accessible hand holds. It's as simple as that!

Yoga Assist

Offers support for greater stretch, grounding, or ease to a safe, clearly aligned pose that is comfortably held by a student with no known applicable injuries

Is performed with firm yet receptive pressure that intentionally directs the tissue along the lines of the pose

Provides directional pressure that follows the lines of stretch or mimics the actions of the pose to accentuate sensations of stretch, grounding, or ease already felt in the pose

Does not aim to change, correct, or advance a pose

I hope that this chapter has helped to convince you, the yoga instructor, why it's important that we start differentiating the ways we describe the types of touch we provide in the classroom. Adjustments and assists both play an important role in the practice, but the two are very different. When we start defining touch clearly in the classroom, this further supports autonomy and personal agency for our students because they know how and why they're being touched and what they're consenting to.

3

LEARN TO READ
THE TISSUES

I was raised by a massage therapist, and therapeutic touch was a mainstay in our household. As an adolescent, I sometimes used my mom's table to give my friends full-body massages. In turn, my mom would often ask to swap massages, and she would always provide feedback about my touch and technique. Unbeknownst to me, I had been getting an education in reading body tissues for most of my life.

When I decided to become a yoga instructor and provide others with similar techniques that helped me heal, I was determined to offer energetically and anatomically safe touch in my classes. I spent years creating, experimenting with, implementing, and honing this methodology for safe, anatomically informed hands-on assists that can be applied by various kinds of teachers to various kinds of students. Students and teachers alike would comment on how different my assists felt and how I needed to teach the technique to a larger audience.

Teaching hands-on yoga assists in my first 200-hour yoga teacher training (YTT) proved more challenging than expected. I had taken for granted how much I already knew about reading and listening to the tissues of the body when I offered touch to someone; I had been learning and practicing it for most of my life. Teaching the methodology to others turned out to require far more than offering stances and techniques. It was vital that my teachers in training learned how to listen to and read the tissues of the body so that they could adapt their touch to each student to help ensure their students' comfort and safety. Being able to read tissues is fundamental to an assist being anatomically safe.

RUBBER BAND THEORY

As both a student and an educator, I have always found analogies helpful to teach something new and complex; we can take something accessible that we are familiar with and liken it to something that is seemingly more complex and unfamiliar to us. In this case, I likened the tissues of the body and their response to stretch to that of a rubber band. From this, the Rubber Band Theory was born, and I started to use it as an approachable way for trainees to learn the somewhat complex task of listening to and reading the tissues of the body.

Being able to listen with your hands is central to offering Rubber Band Method® (RBM) hands-on yoga assists. Although RBM offers a system of stances and techniques that can be repeated from person to person, every body is different, and the RBM teacher must know how to adapt their touch to each individual's unique tissues. This is not a system of assisted stretching that we *do* to our students; it is a collaboration of our technique combined with the unique density of the student's tissues, their individual range of motion, their inherent ability to stretch, their past injuries, and so on. When we know how to listen to the tissues and take the feedback to guide the assist, we are collaboratively offering an assist that is anatomically safe for each unique student.

After successfully training many teachers on how to offer assists from the viewpoint of the Rubber Band Theory, I came to realize that the Rubber Band Theory is at the heart of this system, and so it got its name based on its heart, the Rubber Band Method®.

MUSCLE TISSUE AND FASCIA

Before learning how to read the body's tissues, it's helpful to understand the structure of these tissues. Muscle is the aspect of the body that provides stretch—it is the tissue we are each familiar with being able to palpate, push, and pull. On its own, muscle tissue can stretch a great deal. However, muscle is inextricably linked to fascia, which doesn't stretch quite as much. Every single muscle, down to its individual fibers, is wrapped several times in fascia, giving it structure and a limit to how much it can stretch. Each of these individually wrapped muscle fibers called the endomysium is then bundled together and wrapped again in fascia called the *perimysium*. These fascia-wrapped bundles of individually wrapped muscle fibers are called *fascicles*. These fascicles are then bundled and wrapped again by fascia called the *epimysium* to form a group, or what we call a muscle (e.g., the biceps brachii in the upper arm). All that wrapping is just for each of the muscles! On top of that, we have subcutaneous fascia (found directly under the skin; also termed *superficial fascia*) that sweeps the whole body, like a full-body fascia wrapping. Moreover, certain regions are covered with extra-thick fascia called *aponeurosis* to provide even more protection and limit stretch. Fascia is found throughout the body and is inextricably linked to aspects of practice that we attribute to muscles in yoga, such as range of motion and stretch.

The Rubber Band Theory

Soft tissues have varying degrees of stretch and resistance.

The body is like a rubber band; it can be stretched a great deal, but too much can make it break.

Like a rubber band, once stretched, the body will snap back to its original shape.

Soft Tissues Have Varying Degrees of Stretch and Resistance

The many layers of fascia dictate our range of motion and what we sense as tight or open because of what fascia is composed of. Fascia's constituent parts can restrict (or resist) movement, allow for movement, and either create glide between neighboring structures or adhere neighboring structures together. When adhered layers of fascia stop gliding as they should, the adhesions further affect the felt sense of ease in the tissues, the range of motion they demonstrate, and how much they can stretch.

Fascia comprises collagen, elastin, and ground substance. Collagen fibers limit how much fascia can stretch; collagen creates the feeling of pulling back in the tissues, or what I refer to here as *resistance*. These fibers act like plastic to create form, rigidity, and bounds. More collagen fibers in a region (e.g., iliotibial [IT] band or tendon) equals less stretch, indicating areas where we must be more cautious with stretching. Areas with fewer collagen fibers (e.g., most muscle bellies) will comparatively have more stretch. Elastin, conversely, gives fascia a certain amount of stretch. What keeps fascia nourished and able to glide, stretch, and move is ground substance, a viscous fluid that hydrates the tissue and acts as a sort of lubricant. These three elements affect fascia's ability to create range of motion in our tissues and help to set the bounds for how far tissue can stretch.

Fascia acts like a web that wraps itself around the muscles to help provide strength and support. With repetitive movements, such as 108 sun salutations every month (or weekend!), several vinyasas in every yoga class, or the movements involved in running or weight-lifting, the body builds more collagen fibers in its web to establish greater and greater stability in the regions affected by the repetitive movements. When the collagen builds up in targeted areas within the figurative web, it can affect the overall range of motion and the degree to which a body can stretch (considering all ranges of motion in all planes). This is why we see such variability between body builders and gymnasts, between children and adults, between one yogi and the next; the fascia in our bodies adapts and builds itself to support us in whatever we do most frequently. Because of the activities we have participated in, the sports we have played, the injuries we have sustained, and the lifestyle we choose to practice, we all have different physical histories. Therefore, we are not all built the same in terms of flexibility, stability, and the density of our fascia.

Because all students' tissues are unique to themselves, we must consider each student's tissues in every assist we make. This may initially seem daunting, but it isn't when you know what cues to listen for. Think of each assist like a conversation; is it a conversation if you are the only one talking? No, we would call that a lecture. In a conversation, one person speaks, and the other person listens and *responds*. The point when giving an assist is to listen to the cues you're receiving from the student's tissues and adapt the firmness and strength of your pressure to respond to the information you're receiving. As instructors, we come to the assist with knowledge of the stance to take and the technique to use, but we listen to our student's tissues and adapt our pressure in a way that acknowledges what we hear.

For example, when the body presents its bounds for the stretch (becomes taut and then pulls back), we recognize those signals and pause the directional pressure of the assist so as not to go too far and overstretch the student. Bounds are set by collagen; areas that have more collagen fibers (e.g., the midsection or IT band) will respond quickly and with little amounts of directional pressure. However, collagen is present throughout the body, so interpreting the cues of stretch for each region within each student is a must.

RBM assists employ a technique that includes an anchor and a stretch. Having both an anchor point and a stretch point allows the teacher to understand which tissues they are affecting—and thus reading—in the assist. One point provides the anchor, pinning the tissue in place. The other point provides the stretch, applying directional pressure along the lines of the pose. The teacher is reading the tissues between the anchor and stretch points. Let's look at a few examples.

In child's pose spinal lengthening, the anchor tool is one hand on the sacrum, rooting the student's pelvis downward, and the stretch tool is the opposite hand pressing along the length of the spine toward the crown of the head. The tissues you are listening to for a stretch run along the spine, and you specifically feel them between your two hands, between the anchor and stretch placements.

In supine twist, the anchor tool is on the student's chest, gently pressing the chest to the floor, and the stretch tool is on the student's greater trochanter (hip bone), actively pressing the hip inferiorly toward the feet. The tissues you are listening to for a stretch run along the lateral line of the torso, or between the outer hip and armpit, and you specifically feel them between your two hands, between the anchor and stretch placements.

Points of Contact as Tools

Throughout the technique pages, you'll see me refer to various parts of your hands as tools. This comes from my massage therapy background, from which I learned that we can use our hands and arms in different ways to affect the tissues in various ways. For example, the pressure from a thumb versus an elbow affects tissue very differently, and we can therefore consider them different tools.

As it applies here, we're also changing which parts of our hands we're contacting the student with to best complement the pose and assist. For example, in one assist, we may emphasize pressure in one portion of the palm, and in another, we may use the fingers instead of the palm. In more advanced assists, we recruit other parts of our bodies to provide the anchor and stretch, for example, the feet or knees. Thus, it's applicable to call each point of contact with the student, whether it's the fingertips, palm, base of the thumb, foot, or knees, a "tool" because the device for anchoring and stretching changes from assist to assist. If the tool is grounding the student, it's the anchor tool. If the tool is dynamically applying pressure along the lines of the pose, it's the stretch tool.

Sometimes both hands work to apply the stretch because some part of the student's body is already acting as the anchor. Let's use a couple of examples to illustrate which tissues you'd be listening to and reading in different assists.

In downward dog front press, the student's hands act as the anchor point, and your hands on their hips, lifting up and back, provide the stretch point. The tissues you are listening to run along the lateral side, or outside, of their body, from the pinky finger to the hip crease. This is the line of tissue between the anchor and the stretch—their hands (anchor) to your hands at their hips (stretch).

In corpse-pose leg lift, you aren't looking for a stretch; that's not the purpose of this assist. However, knowing that the student's hips and torso are the anchor point and your hands at the ankles are the stretch point, you know that you're reading the tissues between these points to ensure a stretch does not occur. When lifting the legs, you limit the height to limit the stretch; you're listening to ensure that you don't feel any cues of stretch from the backs of the student's legs or their posterior chain.

Finally, the opposite is also true; sometimes you are providing the anchor as the student lengthens their body along the lines of the shape to provide the stretch. Providing only the anchor can be more nuanced because the student will determine how far they want to take the stretch. Let's look at examples where you are listening to the tissues as the anchor.

In child's pose sacral press, the anchor tool is either one or both of your hands, grounding the student's sacrum and pelvis down toward the floor. The nuance of providing the anchor is that there is a small distance between where the student rests in the pose and where they are anchored; however, the cues of stretch are the same. As you press the sacrum from resting or neutral to the anchored position, you listen for where their body naturally stops, or where the tissues begin to resist. We'll go into more depth on cues of stretch in the next section.

In locust-pose foot anchor, you provide the anchor with both of your hands placed on the balls of the student's feet. The point isn't to force their feet into the floor. Instead, it's to provide enough anchoring pressure to resist the student lifting their feet. This is true of most assists that provide only an anchor; you're providing just enough pressure to keep them anchored rather than blindly forcing their feet into the ground.

The Body Is Like a Rubber Band; It Can Be Stretched a Great Deal, but Too Much Can Make It Break

When you stretch soft tissue—in this case, fascia and muscle, known collectively as *myofascia*—it often feels remarkably like stretching a rubber band. Some tissues stretch easily, others feel denser or more resistant, just like the wide variety of rubber bands out there: some thin and flexible, others thick and unyielding. Each body, like each rubber band, has its own texture, tension, and limit.

A great way to understand the strength and stretch of myofascia is to compare it to a rubber band. When stretching a rubber band, you can likely sense a few things: when there is some slack or give, when there is moderate stretch, and when you have pulled it toward its maximum stretch or breaking point. I think it's safe to assume that at maximum stretch, we can sense that pulling any farther would cause the rubber band to break (who doesn't squint and turn their head when a rubber band gets overstretched?).

The cues a rubber band gives when stretched are like the cues provided by myofascia. If there's no stretch at all, the tissue feels slack. As the tissue begins to become taut, the stretch has begun. Consistent pressure at this point reveals the tissue's edge—a denser, more resistant quality where the myofascia begins to pull back towards its center. This is the optimal amount of pressure in an assist: enough to lengthen the tissue without pushing beyond its natural boundary. Pushing much past this point brings the tissues to maximum stretch, and you risk breaking tissue fibers. Remember that each body has variable amounts of stretch across different regions, and we all have unique limits before soft tissue becomes damaged or breaks like an overstretched rubber band. It is essential that we learn to listen for the cues and understand what they mean before ever getting to that point.

Let's look at the cues a rubber band gives when you stretch it. When you pull a rubber band open, ask yourself what you are sensing or hearing.

- Start with your fingers together and each end of the rubber band near one another. When you immediately begin to pull the rubber band apart, do you sense slackness? Notice how the rubber band moves quickly?

- As soon as the rubber band becomes taut, do you sense some stretch? Notice how the movement immediately slows down?
- Maintain this pressure and stretch slightly farther. Do you notice the rubber band start to resist the pressure or pull back—like the rubber band is trying to pull itself back toward the center?
- Attempt to stretch the rubber band a little farther. Do you notice that it's not as easy to stretch the rubber band and that you would have to use more strength and pressure to get the rubber band to stretch farther?
- You can feel this tactile progression of cues from the rubber band as you increase the stretch from no stretch to maximum stretch. The degree between these points is often minimal, and change occurs quickly, which is why we always move slowly to ensure we sense the varying degrees of stretch our touch intervention is imposing.

The cues you sense and feel from the rubber band when stretched are markedly similar to the cues given by myofascia. Let's use the cues from the rubber band example to see how similar cues show up in assisting:

- Upon immediately applying pressure to your student's tissues, there is a sense of slack or give in the movement of the tissues.
- The tissues seem to move easily and quickly until the slack is taken up between the anchor and stretch placement, and then the movement in the tissues slows down. The tissues become taut, signaling to you that the tissues are being stretched.
- Carefully and slowly, maintain the same pressure and continue directional pressure to feel where the tissues start to pull back toward the anchor or feel as though they are resisting more stretch. This feels like a stopping point in the tissues or a dense edge. This is the boundary.
- At this boundary, it would require more effort and strain to push past this stopping point or dense edge. If you find yourself against this dense edge, trying to press or push past it, you have pushed past the safe bounds of the student's tissues.

When giving an RBM assist, you always want to apply pressure slowly so that you can read the subtle cues from the student's tissues. With your hands, you are sensing a slowing down, a tightening or tautness in the tissues, a bit of resistance as you apply pressure; these are all cues that you have created stretch. At some point, you will sense that you have reached a boundary that feels as though you would need to apply more pressure to get past it; this is the student's boundary of safety. To avoid injury to the tissues, it is at this boundary that we pause or back off the pressure a little rather than providing more pressure. These are all examples of listening to the tissues and then reading the signals you hear.

Finding the Boundary

When you apply the assist slowly, you will often notice that the soft tissue moves easily between the anchor and stretch placements. Rather quickly, with little directional pressure applied, you will notice how the tissue slows down in its movement and becomes taut. Shortly after this point, maintaining the same directional pressure, there is a feeling that the tissue is starting to resist, or there is a bit of density to the tissues. At this point, you would have to increase the pressure of the assist if you were to take your student's tissues farther. *That's the boundary.* Stop when you reach this dense edge to avoid hurting your student. As another way of considering it, you stop when you feel tension in the tissue. Up to and at this point, the assist is helpful. Past this point, the assist can be hurtful.

Please don't concentrate your energy on worrying that you won't sense this boundary. If you're choosing to learn one assist at a time and paying attention when your hands are on a student, moving slowly and listening for cues, you'll feel the boundary of the tissues very clearly. As you learn this technique, I encourage you to check in with your practice partner to help confirm what you sense is the boundary. *Let your practice be your grounds for affirming what you are reading in the tissues.* Assisting requires humble confidence; let your practice instill this in you.

Not listening to your student's tissues and just going through the steps of the technique ignores the unique needs of the person you are touching and can lead to tissue injury. To hurt your student, you must ignore the boundary and forcibly apply pressure past the clear boundary their body has given you. I encourage you to consider assisting as an invitation granted and not a right. This, for me and hopefully for you, is all the more reason why we always approach our students collaboratively from a place of receptive listening.

Just like rubber bands have various sizes, shapes, and amounts of elasticity, this is also true of the different regions within the body and for each yoga student. For example, certain regions of the body contain more collagen and therefore have a greater limit to stretch. If you were to blindly assist these regions without carefully listening to the cues from these tissues, it would be easy to overstretch your student and injure the tissues. For example, the IT band, the abdominal aponeurosis, and the thoracolumbar fascia are all regions with denser collagen; thus, we need to take greater care when offering an assist in these areas. In fact, I've saved most assists that target these regions for the more advanced volumes of the Rubber Band Method® because of the care that is necessary in collagen-dense areas.

Just like we must adapt our touch based on the feedback we receive from the various regions within the body, regions won't feel the same from student to student, and we must adapt our technique. One student's tissues will feel vastly different from another's; therefore, one size or stretch does not fit all. In RBM, the goal is to learn how to listen with your hands, which, in essence, is learning to read the "rubber band nature" of each student's myofascia. Listen with your hands to find where the stretch is, and stop when you feel a slowing down of the tissue movement or the point where the tissues stop easily gliding and begin to pull back, a dense edge. I list various ways to interpret cues from the tissues because we all interpret what we feel with our hands differently. This is why it's important to practice reading the tissues with several different colleagues or friends before bringing the assists into your classroom.

Try This

Gather a few different kinds of rubber bands from office supplies or from the food items you buy. Hopefully, you have rubber bands of varying lengths and thicknesses. I like to close my eyes when doing this exercise so that I can focus on listening with my hands, but you can also do it with your eyes open.

Do This With Each Rubber Band

Pinch the rubber band with each index finger and thumb. Determine which hand will be the static anchor and which hand will be the dynamic (moving) stretch. Begin by bringing your two sets of fingers together; the rubber band will be slack. Slowly begin pulling the stretch fingers away from the anchor, and note the various cues you sense from slack to stretch to dense edge.

Practice sensing the bounds of each rubber band and noting how they are uniquely different. Length doesn't necessarily dictate stretch. Thickness doesn't always dictate density. This also goes for our students; how a body looks doesn't always equal what you will find in its tissues. *Safety note: Be careful not to overstretch and get snapped by the rubber band!*

After you have done this with your index fingers, if your rubber bands are big enough, place both hands inside of each rubber band and repeat the exercise, using each hand rather than only two fingers. Our index fingers and thumbs are very sensitive. Thus, by using the whole hand, you are recruiting more tactile awareness skills. This is the same tactile awareness you will need when touching your students. How do the bounds of the rubber band feel now as compared with using only the index finger and thumb?

I suggest you go back and read through the progressive cues of stretch at the start of this section as you work with each rubber band to feel their different qualities. See if you can sense and interpret the various stages of stretch with your fingers and your hands with the different kinds of rubber bands.

This is a great exercise to hone your tactile sensing skills and learn to listen with your hands. Remember to move slowly in and out of the stretch, even with your rubber bands.

Like a Rubber Band, Once Stretched, the Body Will Snap Back to Its Original Shape

Just as we must take care to move slowly into the assist, we must take equal care to move slowly out of the assist. Moving slowly into the assist allows us to keep our students safe by giving us time to read the subtle cues from their tissues. Moving slowly out of the assist ensures the elastic nature of the student's tissues doesn't cause them to recoil when returning to their original resting position.

Going back to our example of a stretched rubber band, if you were to simply let go of the rubber band once stretched, it would snap back to its original resting shape. The body is the same. Once stretched, the body will quickly recoil back to its original resting position. When you observe an RBM assist, it doesn't appear as though much has changed in the pose. However, the student's myofascia has been stretched to its comfortable bounds. If you were to simply let go without releasing your pressure gradually and slowly, the student's tissues would quickly recoil to the position in which they were resting before the assist.

I call this quick, jarring return or recoil to the resting position the *snapback*. I make a point to demonstrate the snapback in my trainings because it's palpable to all who witness it. Again, it doesn't look like much has happened when you've slowly applied an RBM assist, but if you were to release your hands quickly, the student would bounce back to their original position. For example, if you were to apply the anchor in child's pose sacral press and then quickly release your hands, the student's hips would shoot up (sometimes even bounce a little bit) as they return to where they were before you pressed on them.

The snapback might seem harmless, but does a jarring release support the meditative aspect of yoga practice? No, and our aim is for any touch intervention to serve and support the practice. Therefore, causing the snapback turns the assist into a hurtful touch.

Another example, which I demonstrate very carefully because it's easy to fall over, is releasing the hips after finding the bounds of stretch in downward dog front press. When watching the assist, the shape visually changes very little, but you can see the tissues all along the sides of the student's body jolt down toward their hands and the floor when their weight is quickly released. It isn't injurious to the student, but it is jarring to their practice, so it's considered hurtful touch.

Always enter an assist slowly to listen for the subtle cues of stretch, and always exit an assist slowly to avoid the jarring snapback.

Try This: The Snapback

Child's pose sacral press can provide a very telling demonstration of the snapback. Be sure that whomever you're practicing this with knows that you're aiming to observe the snapback and that the exit will feel jarring. With your willing participant, after applying the anchoring pressure to their sacrum for a few moments, quickly remove your hands. You'll watch their hips pop up and the tissues recoil. This is the snapback and is precisely what we're aiming to avoid by backing out slowly from an assist.

Try This

Recruit one more friend to participate in the previous snapback exercise. Rotate each person through the roles of teacher, student, and observer. Experiencing the snapback from these three vantage points will help reinforce the importance of entering and exiting slowly while also understanding the rubber band–like nature of myofascia.

4

THE RUBBER BAND METHOD® TENETS OF ASSISTING

Now that you understand how to read the tissues when assisting, let's look at the 10 rules to follow when offering assists to help ensure they're energetically and anatomically safe. I call these 10 rules *tenets* because each one helps to ensure your safety and that of your students, and helps to ensure that the assists you provide are helpful and not hurtful.

1. ALWAYS ASK PERMISSION

The first and most important tenet is to always, *always* get permission before assisting your students. The rest of the tenets become irrelevant if a student declines touch because hands-on assists are always optional. For touch to be energetically safe—both mentally and emotionally—it must be consensual. Students need to feel as though they are inviting and agreeing to the touch they receive. Therefore, permission must be obtained before an instructor offers hands-on guidance.

Feeling safe is at the core of our well-being. Whether we realize it or not, we're always gauging our surroundings—consciously or subconsciously—interpreting cues that tell us if we're safe (comfortable, calm) or not (uncomfortable, anxious or even fearful). When we don't feel safe, a stress response is triggered to help protect us. On the other hand, when we feel safe, we can literally breathe easier, think more clearly, and engage with the world in a calmer, more present way. The safety instinct is hardwired into our nervous systems; it shapes how we move through life, how we connect with others, and how we experience the present moment. Touch is such a powerful intervention that it immediately triggers the safety instinct within us, eliciting feelings of safety or lack thereof.

Yoga classes are often perceived as safe spaces, and a well-intended instructor might assume that students inherently feel safe in their class. This assumption can lead to the belief that, because an instructor means well, their touch will be received as safe by every student. But that's simply not the case. As teachers, we cannot know what each individual brings to their mat. This is why, as a Rubber Band Method® (RBM) instructor, it's important to recognize that touch is powerful and experienced uniquely by each person, especially for those who have a history of trauma related to touch or trauma in general.

RBM is not a trauma-informed yoga teacher training. However, it teaches hands-on instructors to be *trauma-sensitive*, which means acknowledging the high probability that in any given class there are likely students who have experienced trauma and may be more sensitive to touch. Trauma-sensitive instruction does not mean eliminating touch; rather, it means offering it in a way that supports students' agency and respects each student's boundaries and unique emotional experience.

In my personal experience, statistics around sexual assault and abuse feel incomplete. Among the many individuals who have shared their stories of trauma with me, only one told me they reported their assault. Traumatic experiences involving touch are often associated with feelings of shame and self-blame, which contribute to under-reporting. However, even with underreporting, data still shows a high prevalence of trauma related to touch. To help illustrate why trauma-sensitive instruction matters, here are some key statistics:

In the United States:

- More than 2 in 5 women (42.0% or 52 million) and more than 2 in 5 men (42.3% or 49.9 million) have experienced physical violence by an intimate partner in their lifetime.[1]
- Almost 1 in 5 women (19.6% or 24.5 million) and 1 in 13 men (7.6% or 8.9 million) have experienced contact sexual violence by an intimate partner in their lifetime.[1]
- 81% of women and 43% of men have experienced some form of sexual harassment and/or sexual assault.[2]
- 1 in 9 girls and 1 in 20 boys under the age of 18 experience sexual abuse or assault at the hands of an adult.[3]

Globally:

- 1 in 3 women (30%) worldwide have experienced physical and/or sexual violence, either from an intimate partner or a non-partner.[4]
- 1 in 8 women and 1 in 11 men were raped or sexually assaulted before the age of 18.[5]
- More than 70% of people worldwide have experienced at least one traumatic event in their lifetime, with an average of 3.2 traumatic experiences per person.[6]

These statistics highlight why a purposeful, consent-based approach to hands-on assists is not just considerate but essential. They underscore the need for trauma-sensitive instruction, reminding us that touch can be deeply personal and, for some, tied to past experiences that shape how it is received. Recognizing this allows us to approach hands-on assists with greater compassion. We cannot always know what each student is bringing to their mat, but the probability that someone in the classroom has experienced trauma—especially trauma related to touch—is high. Knowing this, it becomes clear why obtaining consent before offering hands-on assists is essential.

Yoga is meant to be a space for healing, but healing can only happen when students feel safe. As teachers, we may appreciate hands-on assists, but that doesn't mean our students will. What feels supportive to one student may be distressing to another, and assuming consent simply because someone is in class disregards their autonomy. The simplest way to ensure a safe space? Always ask, always respect the answer, and never assume.

Some teachers may err on the side of caution by assuming a student does not want to be touched and opting not to offer assists. However, I encourage you to never assume that someone does or does not want an assist. If you assume a student does not want to be touched and refrain from offering an assist, they miss out on the opportunity to experience safe touch and to practice agency over their body. For instance, one might assume that individuals from marginalized communities do not want to be touched, but in reality, welcome, safe touch can be deeply healing. Instead of making assumptions, simply ask—and let each student decide for themselves. This approach empowers student agency in the classroom, fosters trust between student and teacher, and helps to ensure that all touch is both safe and consensual.

There are different ways to ask permission. Try to keep in mind that if you ask for a student's permission in front of everyone, they may feel pressured to accept, or they may feel embarrassed to decline if others in the class have accepted. For this reason, one option is to ask for permission after asking everyone to fully or partially close their eyes or after guiding them into a prone (face-down) position. Another great option is to hand out assist coins or cards at the start of class that indicate "I want to be assisted" or "I do not want to be assisted" based on which side of the coin or card is facing up. Students can then place these at the top of their mats to grant their permission for assists. Note that these can be slipping hazards when assisting, so be mindful that your students place the coins or cards on their mats and not on the floor beside them.

I usually ask permission a few minutes into class when everyone's eyes are closed or their heads are facing toward the floor (e.g., in child's pose); I do this with a simple request for a "thumbs-up" or "hand on the belly" if students wish to *decline* hands-on assists. This is important because most students want to receive hands-on assists. If you have to count everyone in the room who wants touch, it's harder to remember who has declined it. Therefore, ask who would prefer *not* to receive hands-on assists. When I use the word *not*, I make sure to annunciate and accentuate that word, such as, "If you wish *not* [pause] to receive assists in your practice today, please give me a thumbs-up." Sometimes, I'll even repeat *not* twice to ensure students haven't misunderstood.

Get Permission First

If you're a hands-on instructor of any kind, whether you're using touch to adjust or assist, I always recommend getting permission right at the start of class. That way, you won't inadvertently touch someone who prefers not to be touched. You'll start the class knowing who has consented to touch.

It's also important to note that assists are always optional, even after students have granted permission. I will say something like, "Please know that assists are optional, and if you wish to decline an assist at any point, just let me know when I approach you." You could also say, "Feel free to wave me off if you'd prefer to decline a specific assist." The point is to communicate with your class. Yes, you are the only one speaking in the room, but communication is also nonverbal, and there are various ways you can communicate back and forth with your students.

If using essential oils (EOs), ask permission to use them even if you have already asked about offering assists in general. When you apply EOs to yourself or others, it's an extra application that needs permission. Some people have sensitivities to EOs and may find them

Suggestions for Asking Permission

Here are various ways you can ask students to communicate their preferences to you regarding touch:

- *Students are in child's pose with arms outstretched toward the top of their mat.* "I'm a hands-on yoga instructor, and I would like to ask permission to provide touch in today's class. I may offer light touch to adjust or correct you, or I may offer a stronger touch to provide assisted stretching. If you'd rather pass on receiving touch, so *no* touch for you, please let me know by giving me two thumbs-ups . . . [wait a few moments]. Thank you [signaling to students that they can relax and stop signaling]."

- *Students are in corpse pose with fully or partially shut eyes at the start of class.* "In my classes, I offer hands-on assists to provide added stretch, grounding, or ease in some of the poses. If you'd prefer *not* to receive assists, please let me know by placing a hand on your belly . . . [wait a few moments to scan the room]. Thank you."

- *Students are in reclined bound angle with fully or partially shut eyes and hands on their bellies at the start of class.* "I'll be offering hands-on assists today to support your practice. This is assisted stretching and is different from an adjustment or correction. If you'd rather *not* receive hands-on assists, please let me know by removing your hands from your belly for a moment [if everyone has their hands on their bellies] . . . [wait a few moments to scan the room]. Thank you."

- *Students are entering the studio or classroom, and you hand them assist coins or cards.* Simply explain to each student that you're a hands-on teacher who sometimes offers light touch to adjust or correct and a stronger touch to assist with added stretch, grounding, or ease in some of the poses. Explain how to show one side of the card or coin to decline and the other side to accept. Also explain that if they change their mind at any point in the practice, they can always switch which side of the card or coin faces up.

bothersome or irritating. For this reason, ask before you use them on your students. When you ask, be specific and state which scent you will be using.

For years, I have used EOs in my corpse-pose neck work. At the start of class, I get permission to provide assists. Near the end of class, when students have just settled into corpse pose, I ask for permission to use EOs; I ask for a "hand to the belly" to decline the assist with EOs. Keeping in mind that all assists are optional, if students decline to receive the assist with EOs, then they decline the assist altogether. This is in no way a punishment to these students; it is how I ensure that I can keep track of those students who do not wish to receive the assist with EOs.

Finally, if a student does decline touch, do not take it personally. I remember a funny incident many years back when one of my regular students declined touch at the start of class. Afterward, she pulled me aside and, with comedic candor, told me that she had such bad gas she was afraid that if I "pushed on her," she'd pass gas! It was a funny moment but also one I could have seriously misconstrued if I had taken it personally. You won't always know why the student has declined assists, but if you use the Rubber Band Method® approach to assists, it is usually safe to assume it has nothing to do with you. However, if all your students are declining assists, it may be a cue to revisit this text and refresh your approach.

2. CHOOSE AN APPROPRIATE STUDENT

Do not offer an assist to a misaligned pose. If the student appears unsafely aligned, is in a different variation of the pose that isn't suitable to assist or is struggling in the pose, do not offer an assist; in most of these instances an adjustment would be better. Only use RBM to assist those students who are safely and comfortably aligned in the shape, who demonstrate the clear lines of the pose to accentuate and offer accessible and secure handholds with which to offer the assist.

To understand this directive, we need to consider what a misaligned shape is. Is it the person in warrior II whose hips are higher than the front knee? Is it someone in downward dog who cannot get their heels to the ground? Or is it the person who uses a prop under their hip in pigeon pose? In fact, none of these examples demonstrates a misaligned shape. What they demonstrate are simple limitations in range of motion with safe, comfortable alignment.

Conversely, a misaligned pose is one where the person looks like they are struggling, there doesn't seem to be integrity through the spine or other joints, or they are in a different variation of the pose that isn't appropriate to assist. Because assists accentuate the lines of the pose, you want to ensure that you're accentuating safe alignment rather than misalignment. Let's look at some examples of students that shouldn't be offered an assist:

- *A student in downward dog has a very long stance, slipping hands, and a rounded spine.* The student is clearly not comfortable. Lengthening their torso would only cause them more struggle; an adjustment would be better.

- *A student is in west-facing pose, or paschimottanasana, with the knees slightly bent, the thighs slightly externally rotated, the spine rounded, and the arms reaching.* This usually indicates a very tight lumbar region or tight hamstrings that would preclude exploring the shape further. An assist amplifies the pose so offering one would not be appropriate here as they are clearly at their limit.

- A student in child's pose has their hips over their knees rather than over the ankles. This is usually an indication of either knee or ankle injury or pain. Though in safe alignment and likely appearing comfortable, this is not a variation of the pose that should be assisted. Adding pressure to the hip region by offering an assist would bring the hips towards the heels, which the student is clearly trying to avoid. Therefore, an assist wouldn't be appropriate on this student as it could cause pain or discomfort.

- *A student is in reclined twist, with the knees more in alignment with the ankles than the hips.* This pose is perfectly safe but is not properly aligned for the assist. When the knees are more aligned with the ankles rather than the hips, it is harder to place a secure handhold on the stretch placement, which is the greater trochanter of the femur. If you don't have a secure handhold with the stretch placement, you run the risk of your hand slipping off, and you could fall on top of the student.

- For purposes of simplicity, when scanning a full room of students, select students who appear to be holding the quintessential expression of the pose, the wide leg child's pose is clearly a wide leg child's pose, or the deer pose is obviously a deer pose. Many students will change the alignment of their pose to accommodate for discomfort, pain, injury, or limited range of motion. This is often a safe expression of tailoring the alignment of the pose to one's personal needs. However, when a student does this, it's an indication that an assist should not be provided to the student. This isn't a matter of exclusion because someone can't "do the perfect pose," but rather a general rule of thumb to help the teacher ensure the safety of their student. We must be selective in the students we choose to assist; if someone isn't appropriate to assist in one pose, simply assist that student in a different pose.

For the assist to be safe for you and the student, it's important that you only offer assists to students who have safe alignment, held comfortably, in the variation of the pose that is appropriate to assist. When a student is safely aligned and in the variation of the pose that can be assisted, the handholds to offer the assist are clear and easily accessible, and the alignment lines of the pose are obvious to follow, allowing you to effectively guide the tissues during the assist. For example, you can't offer a child's pose thigh rotation to a student who has their knees together in traditional child's pose. Similarly, in the recent example of supine twist where the student's knees are more in alignment with their ankles rather than their hips, the handholds aren't suitable to give a safe assist so another student should be selected. Again, it's not a matter of excluding a student because they chose a narrow child's pose or because someone modified their supine twist, but excluding variations of a pose because the handholds are not accessible to offer the assist.

If you are teaching a room full of beginners, it may be difficult to tell when you can give assists because students are generally still learning alignment. Basic assists, such as the chest press or footwork in corpse pose, are a great go-to. Otherwise, if your students do not have any known ankle or knee challenges or injuries, child's pose assists are generally great options too.

When students are in unsafe, misaligned poses, offer an adjustment instead; use verbal cues and possibly light tactile guidance, demonstrate a modification of the pose, or offer a prop to help the student correctly align their body. Again, RBM assists are not appropriate for bodies that are in misalignment.

Even if a student is holding a safely aligned pose comfortably and in the variation accessible for an assist, if they have pain or a known injury, avoid offering assists that require touching or otherwise involve the affected area. For example, if they have a shoulder injury, don't offer bound-angle chest press. If they have a neck injury, avoid corpse-pose neck work. If they have a hip injury, don't offer them child's pose hip press. We modify our asana practice to avoid further hurting an injury; we should do the same when offering assists.

One final thing to consider when choosing an appropriate student is how often you've assisted a student in class. We never want to make student's feel as though they are receiving unwarranted attention that could lead to confusion. When in a class, aim to spread your hands-on attention across the room. That being said, there are a few exceptions. You are never required to assist a particular student or all of your students. I often don't assist new students to my class and never do all of my students receive an assist in a single class if the room is at capacity. However, if I'm teaching a small group, I'll often operate like a typewriter, working from one side of the room to the other; omitting the students who may be expressing variations of the pose that aren't suitable to assist. Obviously, if you're working with private clients who have specifically signed up for one-on-one sessions to receive ample Rubber Band Method® assists during their guided yoga practice, then they'll get all the hands-on attention.

3. YOUR BODY COMES FIRST

RBM teaches six body stances that teachers use when offering assists: high squat, warrior I, low lunge, low squat, kneeling, and easy seat. Teachers provide every RBM assist to the student using one of these six stances (see chapter 7). Using the proper body alignment ensures safety for the teacher and student. The six stances for offering assists ensure that your balance is steady, you are using your legs versus your arms, you are stacking bones whenever possible, you have a straight spine and are not loading your lower back, and you feel strong and stable enough to hold the assist for several breaths.

Always maintain good body mechanics when assisting a student. Remember that assists are optional. If you are uncomfortable, stop the assist and change your stance. Furthermore, if you don't have a solid handhold and feel like you could slip off the student, move your hand or hands and only offer the assist when you do have a solid handhold. Bottom line, if anything feels unsure, unsteady, or insecure, then realign yourself until you feel confident, or don't offer the assist at all. Even if you've already touched the student, if something feels off and you can't correct it, stop what you're doing and slowly step out of the student's space. If it isn't possible to find a safe and comfortable stance to provide the assist, then do not offer the assist. You can easily injure yourself or your student with poor body mechanics.

Remember that assists are always optional. I have attempted to give assists in the past in situations where, because of the proximity of the wall, other students, or some other obstacle, I just could not find a comfortable way to provide them. In such cases, even if I am already in a student's space, I will stop the attempt and exit their space, knowing that I must keep my body safe first. Teachers sometimes feel bad when they can't or don't offer an assist, as if they owe it to the student. I encourage you to let that go and understand that one of your primary intentions is safety for you and your student. Compromising your comfort and stability is compromising safety for you both.

4. HAVE A CLEAR PURPOSE

When offering an assist, both you and your student need to be clear as to its purpose. Become familiar with the purpose of each assist technique before providing the assist to your students. This is like grasping the big picture before getting into the minute details. I've seen teachers get lost in finessing the anchor tool or consumed with trying to read the bounds of tissue because they never paused to consider the big picture. Understand the big picture of each assist first know the alignment of the pose, the anchor and stretch placements, the tissue lines you're reading, and how the assist reinforces the action of the pose. The tools and the respective pieces make sense when you first consider them within the context of the whole.

Each assist technique starts with an explanation of the purpose of the assist. Essentially, the purpose is always to supplement the action of the pose or accentuate the lines of stretch or the experience felt by the student in the pose. Beginning an assist with an understanding of what you're aiming to achieve can help guide where and how to touch your student and how to course correct, if need be, as you become comfortable with reading various body tissues.

Assisting your student with a clear purpose in mind also translates to your students. The student recognizes what you're doing and continues to focus on the felt sense of the pose rather than getting distracted by touch that could otherwise be unclear. When an assist is aligned and in harmony with a student's asana practice, when the assist *assists* the pose, it doesn't detract focus from the practice. In essence, the student's concentration doesn't skip a beat. In fact, purposeful assists add to the focus of the practice because assists create a heightened felt sense of the pose.

If you have no clear purpose for touching your student, the assist will distract them from their practice and can even make them feel a little uncomfortable. When you are touching a student and the purpose is unclear, they will ultimately ask themselves, "Why am I being touched?" If it's not clear to the student why you are touching them, their attention has been pulled from the present moment, and the touch has served to disrupt their practice. As one of my students shared with me, "I never go back to classes where the teacher seems to be touching me just for the sake of touching me. It makes me uncomfortable. I mean, why are they touching me?" I couldn't agree with her more. If you're being touched by your yoga teacher, there should be a clear reason why; both the teacher and student must know the purpose.

5. ENTER AND EXIT SLOWLY

On a simple level, we want to match the energy of our students. Yoga is a moving meditation, and how you enter and exit the student's space, as well as how you touch them, should reflect the student's energy. In this context, *entering* means applying pressure, and *exiting* means withdrawing pressure. It is essential to ensure that you enter and exit an assist slowly to keep the assist safe and helpful to the student. Additionally, throughout the assist—and generally anytime you touch your students—your movements should be slow and steady. Whether you offer touch as an assist or an adjustment, quick movements can be jarring, both physically and mentally.

As explained in chapter 3, Learn to Read the Tissues, each body you touch will be different from the next. Because of this, you must adapt the pressure and depth of each assist by reading the cues from the tissues. If there are no anomalous cues (pops, grinding, etc.), you will enter slowly to feel for when the tissues become taut or begin to stretch. When you sense the tissues somewhat resisting or pulling back, you've found the bound of the stretch. You're listening or feeling for this bound, or dense edge, so that you can pause the pressure and hold the pressure at that bound for a few moments or breaths. Then, you'll back out of the assist slowly and guide the student's tissues back to their natural resting position.

You won't be able to pick up on anomalous cues unless you're entering slowly. With anomalous cues, you need to tune in and discern what's going on. Is there a pop or grind? If so, pause there; don't offer more pressure. You might ask the student whether the pressure is comfortable. As another example, if you've applied what feels like standard pressure or stretch to the tissues but you aren't sensing any tautness or feedback from the student's tissues, pause again. Is this person hypermobile, or do they have hyperflexible tissues? Or do you have your anchor and stretch placement wrong and need to correct your handholds? Or perhaps you've applied pressure to a student, and the tissues feel like a dense rock. Your first instinct might be to press harder. Instead, pause. Listen more intently to the cues from their tissues; they might not need more pressure, but more time for the tissues to respond. In all these situations, you're going slow enough to pick up on the cues from the tissues and adapting your touch accordingly.

Exiting slowly is just as important as entering slowly. In the discussion of the Rubber Band Theory in chapter 3, we learned that myofascia responds to stretch a lot like a rubber band. Once the tissue is stretched, it'll quickly recoil if released abruptly. This jarring recoil is the snapback. The snapback isn't comfortable for the student, so you must always exit slowly to avoid it. Be sure to back out slowly and guide the tissues to their original resting position before releasing your handhold and stepping out of the student's space.

6. USE FIRM, DIRECTIONAL PRESSURE

Have you ever had someone attempt to deepen the stretch in your pose, but you could barely feel their touch? Have you had someone press on you, and it felt like hard, uncomfortable jabs? Or have you ever received a massage and thought, "Oh, that's nice, but wait, why is my yoga teacher massaging me?" These are all examples of unhelpful assists because of the poor quality of touch. With poor-quality touch, the student gets pulled from their practice by thinking about the instructor's touch—to the student, the touch may seem pointless, painful, or inappropriate. With good-quality touch, students will interpret your assists as purposeful and helpful.

Use a Firm Touch

We don't touch our students just to place our hands on them. The point is to add something to their practice. Firm touch uses enough pressure to "hook into" or "sink into" the tissue in order to guide the tissues somewhere, slowly. In contrast, light touch doesn't take the tissue anywhere; it doesn't guide it into a stretch.

Whenever you place your hands on a student, you must ensure that you have a good handhold before attempting the assist. You will find a good handhold by slowly sinking your hand into the tissues. Applying enough pressure to sink into the tissues is considered firm pressure.

A Firm Touch Is Receptive but Strong and Never Forceful

Simply put, firm touch means you are sinking into the student's tissues enough to have a handhold. You are not grabbing, squeezing, or forcing. If you notice you are doing any of these or you are applying a lot of effort to give the assist, you are being too forceful.

I had a trainee who was naturally good at giving assists, but her ongoing challenge was understanding the meaning of "firm but receptive." When she provided assists, she had all elements of the technique in place; she understood the purpose and had the stance, handholds, and lines of the shape down. However, whenever she offered an assist, it felt too firm, as if her hands were painfully jabbing into my tissue. Her touch felt forceful and jarring rather than supportive.

I tried every adjective I could to describe how to soften her hands, but nothing was translating for her. Eventually, I said, "Keep the strength of your assist, but imagine that you are giving this assist to your child." Instantly, her hands softened, and her assist felt strong but receptive. Her touch was firm while also feeling supportive and nurturing. What she then understood was the receptivity that we need to use when offering an assist. It's easy to get lost in the technique and forget that we're touching someone, an action that requires genuine receptivity and care.

Try This

Explore a Rigid Palm

When assisting, you want your hands to feel soft rather than rigid. To understand the concept of a rigid hand, spread your fingers and stretch out your palm and hand as much as possible, then use your palm to palpate down the length of your thigh. How does it feel?

Explore a Supple Palm

Now soften your hand. Shake out your hand first, give it a little stretch, and then let your hand feel soft and natural. Place your relaxed hand on your thigh, and lift your fingers away only slightly so that they still lie on your thigh but do not dig in or grab at the thigh; this is only a slight lift or extension of the fingers. Palpate down the length of your thigh and compare how this feels to the rigid palm. Did one feel better than the other?

Use this type of supple palm when offering assists; if your hands feel soft, but strong, your touch will too.

Little Effort Is Required When You Employ the Anchor and Stretch Application

When you use the anchor and stretch application, the anchor will pin one end of the student's body. When you begin to apply firm directional pressure with the stretch placement along the action or alignment lines of the pose, it will take little effort to produce a stretch because the tissue is pinned at its anchor. You will feel the tissues become taut between the anchor and stretch placements (these are the tissues you're reading), signaling that a stretch is occurring. Because this is a subtle movement, the pressure should never be forceful. If you find yourself forcing, then stop the assist.

Don't Be Creepy or Sensual

In general, students don't want to be grabbed or massaged. The most frequently used RBM tools are the palmar surface of the hand, the base of the thumb, or the pinky edge of the hand instead of the fingers. In assists that use the thigh-rotation technique, you will use your fingers, but avoid using your fingertips, which can feel "grabby." In neck work and work involving the feet, we use the tips of the fingers, but we use palpation rather than massaging or grabbing.

To avoid being sensual, never massage a student's body. At all times, we are only using firm pressure to press (long-held pressure), provide traction (lengthening or pulling), or palpate (slow, repeating pressure on and off). If you find yourself grasping at tissues or rubbing the tissues, such as in a circular, stroking motion, you've wandered into massaging and should stop the assist. We don't make sexual advances toward our students, and we never want to lead them to think that we are through our touch.

If You Are Feeling Unsure, Always Check in on the Strength or Pressure of the Assist

In general, you do not want to constantly ask students if your pressure is okay; that pulls them from their practice. You can avoid this by refining your quality of touch with colleagues and friends before offering assists in the classroom. However, if you are unsure in the classroom, ask. Especially when you are first learning, do not be afraid to ask. When asking, be specific: "Is this pressure comfortable?"

7. FOLLOW THE LINES OF THE POSE

All RBM assists reinforce the actions or experience of a pose, accentuate the lines of stretch felt within the pose, or follow the alignment lines of the pose to serve an obvious purpose in the student's practice. The assists mimic the action of the pose (e.g., grounding the feet in locust pose), reinforce the energy of the pose (e.g., deep relaxation in corpse-pose neck traction), or accentuate the stretch already experienced in the pose (e.g., supine twist spinal lengthening).

Teachers must understand the basic alignment of the pose they are assisting so that it's clear what actions or alignment lines they should follow. With an understanding of alignment, it should be relatively easy to see what lines you are following in your student's body as the student holds a pose. However, let's use a few examples to make it clear.

In downward dog, the student isn't pressing their hips to the back of the room, so to assist them in that direction wouldn't feel good to the student. The student is pressing their hips *up* and then *back*, which looks like a diagonal line made from their fingertips to their hips. Follow this diagonal line, lifting up from the ilium (hip bones) and then back.

In child's pose spinal lengthening, the student is lengthening their arms toward the top of their mat. The lines of the pose follow their spine, from the hips to the fingertips. If you attempted to offer an assist along the spine by pressing their spine down into the floor, it would not feel good to the student. The student isn't trying to press their body into the floor, so we shouldn't aim to either. Instead, we follow the lines of the shape and provide directional pressure along the length of their spine toward the top of their mat rather than toward the floor. The pressure applied in the assist mimics the lines of the shape and feels much better to the student than having their shoulders and face pressed into the mat.

In supine twist, most teachers assume that the line of the pose is the direction in which the knees are dropping into rotation. However, I invite you to take the shape and drop your knees to the right. What happened to your left shoulder? It may be subtle or pronounced in your own body, but when you drop your knees in a twist, the opposite side of the torso receives a stretch from hip to shoulder. This line along the outside of the torso, from hip to shoulder, is the line of stretch in this pose. It can be dangerous to force a student's body into rotation, regardless of where the rotation is taking place in the body. In this example, it's the lumbar spine (low back). The student has found their limit to rotation, and we must honor that by not forcing them into a deeper rotation. If you were to anchor your hand on the shoulder and rotate a student's hips deeper into the twist, it would likely feel scary for the student and possibly lead to injury in the lumbar area or lower back. However, if you anchor your hand on the chest and press their hip inferiorly (toward the bottom of their mat or toward their heels), this mimics the lines of stretch created by the shape and will feel very, very good to the student.

Following the lines of the pose requires an understanding of alignment. If you are unsure, you can always practice on a friend or take the shape in your own body to notice in which direction you are lengthening or the actions you are taking to find the pose (e.g., hips to the heels in child's pose) and to feel the lines of stretch (e.g., across the upper back in deer pose) or general energy of a pose (e.g., the grounding in reclined bound angle).

8. DO NOT ASSIST ON SKIN

As a general rule, never place your hands on exposed skin to provide an assist. Nowadays, you will find many students practicing with their shirts off, others in a sports bra, or some in shorts exposing most of the thigh. In all these instances, you would not offer hands-on assists to the exposed regions.

Whether or not the yoga instructor realizes it, in every classroom, there is a power differential that favors the teacher. The teacher is the one leading the room, and the students are following. To ensure we respect our students fully and never misuse or abuse that power differential, we never place our hands on bare skin. We'll talk about a few exceptions to this rule, but generally speaking, avoid touching skin. Simply consider a student with ample exposed skin not suitable for specific assists that would require you to touch their exposed regions.

I remember training a new teacher on the Rubber Band Method® and I had invited her to come assist my class. I introduced her to my class, told them she was practicing her assists, and requested permission for her to offer touch. At the end of class, one of my regular students approached me and complimented the teacher on her general application. However, she said that at one point, my assistant startled her and made her a little uncomfortable when she placed her hands on her bare back. She said it felt "really handsy," and she recommended I talk to the trainee because she had never felt me offer this kind of assist in my classroom before. Of course, the student was right, and I was grateful for the feedback to provide to my teacher in training.

When teachers touch skin, students can easily misconstrue the touch as sensual. Because a power dynamic exists between teacher and student, the boundaries can become confusing and blurry when teachers touch skin. Skin is a vulnerable, intimate part of the body that is usually only touched by people we're intimate with. Consider how often your friends or acquaintances touch your bare back, your waistline, or your bare thigh. It just isn't done in most cultures, so the classroom should be no exception. Respect your students' boundaries and uphold your own when offering assists by not touching skin.

Here are some caveats to working with bare skin. If you can pull down clothing to avoid touching skin, do so to offer the assist. If the clothing has simply shifted to reveal more skin, you can easily pull it down and cover the skin to offer the assist. It's common and customary for me to pull the end of a tank top down when offering a spinal lengthening or pull the end of the student's shorts farther along the thigh before offering a thigh rotation. This is only a slight shift of clothing and does not involve moving someone's top or bottoms entirely. *Avoid moving someone's clothing drastically; a slight shift is okay.*

It is generally acceptable to touch skin in the regions of the arms and shoulders, neck, scalp, and feet. These locations are generally acceptable to touch without cloth covering. However, make sure to respect any cultural preferences among the students in your class regarding touching these bare regions.

You will note that I didn't list the face. I strongly recommend that teachers avoid touching their students' faces in a public classroom setting, including the forehead. Faces are usually sweaty and sometimes covered in makeup or acne, and touching multiple faces in a crowded classroom isn't hygienic (keep in mind how many orifices are on the face). Also, for some, the face is a very vulnerable place to be touched, and it can feel invasive. Therefore, I suggest avoiding touching the face altogether. If you are fond of the idea of ending savasana neck work with a third eye press, I recommend the crown chakra instead to offer a similar ending that avoids touching the face.

9. ALWAYS ASSIST BOTH SIDES

This tenet only applies if there are two sides. In downward dog, for example, there are no sides. This is also true of wide-leg forward fold, child's pose, and bound angle—these asanas do not have two sides. However, reclined twist, deer pose, reverse warrior, janu sirsasana, pigeon pose, and many others have two sides, a right and a left. Because RBM works with lengthening the myofascia, it is imperative that you assist the same student on both sides. This mirrors the fundamental tenet of yoga asana practice: We always practice both sides to keep the body balanced. If we lengthen one side of our student in supine twist and don't assist the other side, they will likely feel imbalanced.

Keep things like obstacles, other students, and walls in mind when offering assists on both sides. For example, avoid choosing the student who is right next to the wall when offering a supine twist assist. Although you can find a comfortable stance on the first side, once they switch sides, you might not be able to find a safe stance beside them.

The issue of occasionally forgetting to assist the second side is worth noting. You know what? It happens! Maybe you are offering alignment cues, are deep into your theme, and are assisting several students simultaneously. When you return for the second side, you suddenly realize you cannot recall all the students you assisted on the first side. Do not fret! If you occasionally make the mistake of only assisting one side, your student will not be physically harmed or impaired in any way. However, they might notice that the side that got missed isn't quite as open as the other side. You can think of it as being similar to forgetting to do both legs in pigeon pose; you feel otherwise fine, but one side feels more open than the other. So, don't worry if you forget, but always aim to assist the same student on both sides of a two-sided asana.

On the subject of forgetfulness, if you frequently forget who you have assisted, only assist one student per pose and wait to assist multiple students in a pose until you can keep track.

10. BE MINDFUL WHEN ASSISTING JOINTS

When working with RBM assists, you will often use bony landmarks to help guide your hand placement; otherwise, you will not intentionally move bones. What the RBM teacher aims to assist is the soft tissue, the myofascia between bony landmarks. When we use bones as handholds (e.g., in downward dog front press), it is to offer support to the soft tissues attached to or between the anchor and stretch placements.

Joints are sites of articulation between bones, so any force placed on these points will cause not only the tissue but also the bones to move. Firm touch can feel unpleasantly intense around the joint region. Lighten the pressure considerably when you work near joints.

The shoulders, knees, and elbows are sites where you want to take the most care when applying firm touch. A few of the assists in this book work near the shoulders. Although we're still using firm, intentional pressure, it is lighter near the shoulder than at the hip. Furthermore, listening with your hands as you come in and out of the assists near the shoulder joints becomes important. Do you sense popping? Too much movement? Stop where you are, and don't go further; less is more here.

As a general rule, do not apply pressure to the kneecap when the student is lying face-up or face-down with their knees extended or straight; this also applies to the elbow joints. For both of these hinge joints, when they are in flexion or bent, you can more safely work near the joint.

The hips are the exception. Generally speaking, you can apply more pressure to the hips. But caution is still warranted; conditions such as hip dysplasia or hip replacements can be aggravated and even reinjured when you apply significant pressure while the student is in asana shapes. This is one reason why RBM-trained instructors ask about injuries, pain, and surgeries at the start of every class. Entering slowly and learning to listen with your hands for the bounds of each student's tissues is also how you help avoid taking tissues or joints too far.

Rubber Band Method® Tenets of Touch

1. Always ask permission.
2. Choose an appropriate student.
3. Your body comes first.
4. Have a clear purpose.
5. Enter and exit slowly.
6. Use firm, directional pressure.
7. Follow the lines of the pose.
8. Do not assist on skin.
9. Always assist both sides.
10. Be mindful when assisting joints.

5
RESPECTFUL ASSISTS

Although providing touch in the yoga setting is yet another technique to amplify the benefits of the practice, such as building in breath work, aromatherapy, meditation, and so forth, you must use it with a serious degree of respect for each student's energetic space and anatomical form. I consider being in a student's space an honorable invite that I must handle with care. I emphasize to all my trainees how important it is to remember that they're touching a living, breathing person who has a mental, emotional, and physical history; our energetic presence in their space and our physical touch interact with what the student brings to the mat, and they have an impact on that person. For this reason, it's imperative that the teacher tune in to their student, treat them with respect energetically and physically, and touch the student as if the teacher is earning the invite to enter their space the next time.

To provide respectful assists, there are many things to consider. First, we'll discuss how to ensure that our touch is helpful and never hurtful. The techniques in this book state the step-by-step how-to of each assist, but there are also general things to consider when you enter a student's space. The last segment looks at how Rubber Band Method® (RBM) assists can be respectfully applied in the context of trauma-informed yoga. This chapter provides tips to help ensure our assists are energetically safe and feel mentally and emotionally safe to the student.

HURTFUL VERSUS HELPFUL TOUCH

In chapter 1, we looked at the science behind the benefits of touch, and as we learned, the benefits are huge! One important takeaway from that chapter is that for touch to be beneficial, it must be consensual. It must become common practice that we, as teachers, tactfully request consent to touch our students; otherwise, there's no solid foundation for touch to be beneficial.

Without explicit consent, there's no way of knowing how touch is being perceived and received by the students. If the touch isn't helpful; if it's unclear or seemingly pointless; or if it feels disrespectful, uncomfortable, or painful, there's no way for the student to opt out of receiving it when consent isn't agreed upon. The only thing the student can do is choose to endure it or stop coming to that instructor's class.

Beyond not requesting and receiving consent, there are many other ways touch can be hurtful. Touch that feels disrespectful, uncomfortable, or even unclear and pointless can create a stress response, which can be physiologically hurtful to the student. Moreover, some touch interventions can be downright injurious; for example, forcing a student's body into yoga shapes can cause tissue damage and injury.

Over decades of practice and countless interviews with trainees and students, I've compiled a simple list that helps identify what kinds of touch are hurtful in the yoga classroom.

Hurtful Touch

Nonconsensual

Serves no obvious purpose in the asana practice

Distracts the student from their practice

Feels disrespectful

Not anatomically informed

Causes physical, mental, or emotional harm

Here are some examples of hurtful touch from my own experience and that of my students and trainees:

- My friend had good levels of flexibility and didn't feel much sensation in downward dog. To find sensation, she would hyperflex her shoulders, pressing her chest exaggeratedly back toward her thighs. The teacher corrected her by grabbing her ponytail and pulling her forward to draw her shoulders out of the hyperflexed position.

- A teacher wanted me to externally rotate or roll my shoulders out more in downward dog, which I wasn't physically able to do to her expectations. She proceeded to grab the heads of my shoulders and forcefully rotate my shoulders outward. It was painful. She only stopped when I dropped my knees and sat up quickly.

- I had a male instructor who was giving me more tactile attention than other students, which alone made me feel uncomfortable. Eventually, he climbed beneath my downward dog to talk to me. He was not at the side but directly underneath me, lying on his back and talking to me in a flirtatious way. I felt cornered and uncomfortable because my boundaries were being crossed, and as his student, I wasn't sure what I could do.

- My friend had a lumbar disc injury but felt comfortable practicing yoga and knew how to practice without aggravating it. He had great thoracic mobility and found reclined twists rather easy. The teacher came over and, instead of lengthening his spine, pushed his hips deeper into rotation; he felt his lower back pop and had lower back pain afterward.

- A teacher grabbed my bound wrists and the back of my head and forcefully pressed my head and hands to the floor in bound wide-legged forward fold. The idea was to force me into the "ideal shape," regardless of whether I wanted to go there or if my tissues were capable of doing so. The assist caused ongoing pain, indicating a likely tissue tear to my anterior (front) shoulder.

- One of my students reported that while she was in corpse pose, the teacher placed her hands on her thighs without warning, startling her and causing her to jump, then proceeded to squeeze her legs from the thighs down to her feet. The student explained she didn't mind her legs being touched, but she felt startled by the unexpected contact.

- After class, my friend explained how the yoga teacher had given him a "very sensual" head massage in corpse pose. He said it felt good, but it was also very confusing and, as a result, distracting.

- A fellow teacher explained her confusion over how the instructor touched her in extended triangle pose. She said the teacher placed one hand on her shoulder and wrapped her index and thumb around the wrist of her extended arm. There was no guidance, correction, or clear intention, she explained; it felt like the instructor was merely touching her just to touch her. This lack of clarity pulled her from her presence in the pose, creating a disruption to the focus of her practice.

- A trainee of mine once shared her experience from another training, where the instructor advised participants to correct students with protracted chins or forward head posture by placing a hand on the student's chin and physically pushing it. She felt this crossed a boundary, violating students' space, even though the instructor insisted it was an appropriate method of correction. If that kind of cue seems harmless at first glance, ask yourself which feels more respectful of your boundaries: having another adult place their hands on your face and push your head back, or seeing the instructor demonstrate drawing the head back by placing their hand on their own chin and retracting their head?

These examples are given to illustrate the various ways hurtful touch shows up in the yoga classroom; some of the examples might not seem hurtful at all, whereas others are obviously hurtful. Ultimately, if we're going to touch our students, we must have permission to do so and *be adding something to their practice.*

This is where having a clear purpose comes in. Touching a student is a touch intervention; we are intervening in our student's practice by touching them. If we're going to do this, if we're going to interrupt their moving meditation, then it needs to *obviously* serve a purpose and add something to the practice. I say "obviously" because it should be obvious to the student how our touch supports them. Does being startled in savasana assist the meditation in this pose? Is wondering why a teacher is touching us adding to the focus of the practice? Is a sensual massage that confuses the student not a betrayal of boundaries? Put simply, hurtful touch is any touch that distracts the student from their practice; touch that causes the student to wonder about the intent of their teacher's touch; and, of course, any kind of disrespectful touch that is not anatomically informed and causes mental, emotional, or physical discomfort or pain.

In contrast, let's review how touch can be helpful for students.

Helpful Touch

Is consensual, with permission discreetly requested and received

Has a clear purpose to enhance or serve the practice in some way

Uses precise hand placement to be safe and effective

Adapts touch with intention—gentle and directive in adjustments, firm but receptive in assists

Helpful touch may not always provoke dramatic reactions (beyond the frequent positive feedback after class), but its impact is often seen in increased student attendance, retention, and referrals. When students experience touch that is consent-based, anatomically informed, and adds something useful to the asana practice, they recognize the difference. It feels good, it feels purposeful, and it invites them deeper into their practice (just like pranayama, bandha, or any other supportive technique). RBM instructors often find that their classes grow quickly, private sessions increase, and students keep returning—not just for the sequencing or cueing, but because the touch they receive feels safe, supportive, and beneficial. Helpful touch communicates care and clarity without words. It builds credibility, fosters connection, and becomes a defining feature of the class experience.

Here are a few examples of helpful touch in the classroom from my own experience and that of my students and trainees:

- I once worked for a wonderful nonprofit organization, the Art of Yoga Project (AYP), that brings yoga and art to incarcerated youths. My years teaching for AYP proved to me that safe touch can be a helpful application for anyone healing from post traumatic stress disorder (PTSD) and that my journey was not unique. In fact, witnessing how the youths responded to the assists (emphatically requesting more) and how the assists benefited the student–teacher relationship overall convinced me that if touch is considered safe to the person receiving it, it is a powerful healing application. (More discussion of RBM and trauma is provided later in the chapter.)

- During the photoshoot for the *Advanced Applications* volume, my assistant was demonstrating king pigeon. Using the RBM assist, I guided her safely into the full expression of this very advanced backbend. She could not believe she could get there! She'd never been able to access this pose before. Her sense of achievement in finding a pose she'd never been able to access fully was infectious and felt by all present. (Please note that I only assisted the pose; she got there on her own. We started with a strap, but after her body received the assist, she went into the full expression of the pose naturally and easily. RBM never aims to force students into more advanced variations of the pose.)

- I have had students over the years come to me privately and thank me for the support and nurturing they received through the helpful touch provided in the classroom that helped them address underlying trauma from assault. There are no words for how meaningful it is to me to offer RBM in a public classroom setting and be able to simultaneously help certain individuals heal from their trauma.

- A student of mine who experienced her first assist in supine twist exclaimed, "Oh my gosh, when you gave me that assist in the twist, it felt so good! Thanks for doing both sides; I didn't realize how different I was from left to right—I really needed it." I have hundreds and hundreds of stories like this. After every single class I've taught, students come up and thank me for the assists they received. I almost always hear, "Those assists felt *soooo* good!" The best part is that students will often report back to me on where and how they felt the assist, demonstrating to me that the purpose of the assists is obvious to my students.

- One of my teacher trainees had this to say about her overall experience with helpful touch:

> The Rubber Band Method® has completely transformed my experience as both a yoga teacher and a student. Learning this method has opened my eyes to the profound impact intentional and purposeful assists and adjustments can have on students during their practice. As a newer yoga teacher, I was eager to offer a more hands-on experience for my students, but I struggled to understand the purpose behind hands-on assistance. When I received assists as a student, it often felt awkward and left me questioning their necessity. Having been in the fitness industry for a long time, I value alignment and the importance of offering purposeful guidance in my classes. When Kiara used the Rubber Band Method® to assist me in a class, I finally experienced what I had been searching for. Her execution of the method was remarkable. Her hands-on approach was confident and intentional, and I could feel the strength, opening, and power coursing through my body with each assist. Her presence felt safe and, in that moment, I knew I wanted to learn from her. Since incorporating the Rubber Band Method® into my teaching, I have noticed my classes

filling up more and receiving positive feedback from my students about the depth the assists bring to their practice. I believe every yoga teacher could benefit from understanding and implementing this methodology, as it has the power to truly enhance the student's experience and create a deeper connection in their practice.

The first and most important element of helpful touch is that it's based on consent; you have asked the student if they want to be touched, and you've given them a discreet way to consent or decline. Consent is crucial in yoga because a power differential that favors the teacher exists in the classroom. This is why it's essential that consent and personal agency become a regular practice in our classrooms: Students must know that they have power over their bodies in this setting too. Consent is the first step in ensuring the touch we offer is beneficial.

For touch to be truly helpful—whether it's an adjustment or an assist—we should always be able to answer three questions: Why are we touching our student? Where are we touching our student? How are we touching our student? In this book, every technique outlines its purpose because understanding why we use touch is essential. Every RBM assist adds something to the student's practice. If you're adjusting a student, the same principle applies: you must know why you're using touch and what you're trying to achieve by changing their pose.

Where we place our hands might be the most important question we must answer when assisting or adjusting. Where ensures the touch is appropriate and serves a clear purpose. That's why each technique page includes an anatomical figure of the yoga pose being assisted. These figures highlight the anchor and stretch placements and illustrate the lines of stretch and myofascial involvement, so you can confidently understand what structures you're influencing with every assist.

Knowing how to touch a student defines the quality of touch. In an adjustment, touch is light, directive, and aimed at guiding the student toward more supportive alignment. In an assist, touch is firm while also being receptive, allowing the pressure to adapt to the student's unique body and myofascia. A truly helpful assist takes more than just applying pressure—it requires the ability to read the student's body tissues and respond to the cues they express. This adaptability ensures that touch remains supportive rather than forceful.

When we understand why, where, and how to use touch, we better ensure that every intervention is helpful rather than harmful. Safe touch, offered with respect for a student's agency and physical boundaries, can be transformative. It narrows the divide between self and other, builds trust, and reinforces personal agency. Students discover new possibilities in their bodies, and genuine healing begins.

This is helpful touch.

HOW TO BE IN A STUDENT'S SPACE

You want to add to the student's experience, not detract from it. I think of being in someone's space as an invitation to respect and honor. When I approach a student using this mindset, I naturally seem to take extra care, and I hope all teachers employing the RBM will be mindful to do the same.

There are many things to consider when you are stepping into a student's space. In a way, the yoga mat acts as your student's little island of autonomy within the classroom, so you must be considerate when entering that space. These considerations are discussed next, beginning with being *fully* in your student's space.

Never Reach; Be Fully in Your Student's Space

When first learning to offer assists, many yoga instructors are timid about being in the student's space. Being timid or unsure results in the teacher avoiding getting too close to their student and having to reach to touch the student. If you are reaching, you are not fully in your student's space. Furthermore, by reaching, the teacher is not well equipped to give a safe assist because the stance is inherently compromised. If you are going to offer assists, you must be confident enough to be in your student's space.

You know you are fully in your student's space when you can touch your student while maintaining a comfortable stance. When in a comfortable stance, you use the strength of the legs rather than the arms, you can maintain a straight spine throughout the assist, your shoulders are often stacked over or behind the wrists, your balance is steady, you feel comfortable, and the action of the assist requires marginal effort.

Helpful Touch From a Place of Stability

Touch needs to be helpful for all involved. Assisting from a stable stance ensures that we won't misalign our student, knock them off their balance, or fall on top of them. What is of equal importance, is that we don't sacrifice our bodies to do this. I created RBM after experiencing an injury when assisting a student who was considerably larger than me. A stable stance is like a stable base in yoga. When we build the alignment in our poses, we start from our base. The teacher, in effect, is the base of the assist. How the teacher is holding themselves creates either a steady or unsteady assist. If the teacher makes sure that they are steady before ever touching their student, the assist can be a helpful one.

Never Surprise a Student With Your Touch; Let Them Know You're There by Rubbing Your Hands Together, If Needed

Usually, the student will know when you have stepped into their space to offer an assist, but not always. If you are offering assists in a restorative class or in corpse pose, the student might not know you are there, and touching them could be startling. If you have quietly entered your student's space and they appear to be in a state of internalization or meditation, rub your hands together before you touch the student. The soft brushing of the hands will subtly alert the student that you are at their mat and about to touch them. It's also a very gentle, inviting sound that is less invasive than an unanticipated assist.

When Working Close to the Student's Face, Avoid Breathing Directly on Them

Be mindful not to breathe on the student's face. Breathing on the student is especially easy to do when the student is in corpse pose or any other floor pose where the student is supine (facing up) and you are close to or above their face. Turn your head slightly to direct your breath away from them.

If You Have Cold Hands, Warm Them Before Touching Your Student

Some teachers often have cold hands. If this applies to you, rub your hands together and warm them up before touching your students; cold fingers on a warm neck or shoulder creates an uncomfortable sensation.

Be Mindful of the Transition

Accidentally touching sensitive areas is a bigger risk when coming into or out of a pose. For this reason, be mindful of how you are transitioning in and out of the student's space. If you are pressing on the hips, be careful not to brush or touch the genitals or the groin region. If you are working around the shoulders, be careful not to brush or touch the breasts. If you take care to enter slowly and exit slowly to avoid the snapback, it will be easier to avoid grazing sensitive areas as you also slowly step out of a student's space.

Sometimes, when we take care to avoid our students' sensitive areas, we forget about our own. Be mindful not to put your pelvis or breasts in the student's face or on any part of their body. This unfortunate occurrence can easily happen when giving assists on the floor, especially in supine twist. Try to keep some distance between your sensitive regions and the student's face and body. Consider keeping a barrier between your sensitive areas and the student's head too. For example, in supine twist, your anchor arm can act as a barrier, and in corpse-pose neck traction, your crossed legs act as a barrier.

Be Conscious of Odors and Aromas

Last but not least, be mindful of your hygiene. Because assists require that you be fully in your students' space, ensure that you are free of any distracting body odors that may feel invasive to your students. Additionally, avoid any strong perfumes, oils, or fragrances that might also seem invasive to a sensitive person. If you use essential oils, request permission before bringing them into the student's personal space.

RUBBER BAND METHOD®
AND TRAUMA

The Rubber Band Method® is intended for use in public yoga classes. My experience with PTSD and training in trauma-informed yoga led me to create an approach to touch that was sensitive to the undisclosed or unacknowledged trauma that may be present in any public classroom. This is why the methodology is grounded in consent while also being anatomically informed, or what I refer to as *energetically and anatomically safe.*

RBM is *not* a trauma-informed yoga training. However, because I've designed it to be fundamentally safe for undisclosed trauma in a public class setting, it can just as easily be adapted as a tool for use by qualified instructors of trauma-informed yoga. In our asana practice, we modify poses for students with a physical injury. With assisting, we do the same. When students have physical injuries, we avoid certain assists to avoid aggravating the injury. Trauma is a mental and emotional injury that deserves the same respect as a physical injury. Instructors ought to avoid certain assists to ensure no retraumatization or triggering occurs (more on this later in the chapter).

I'm including this section on RBM and trauma because the overall intention is to set the standard for safe touch in yoga classrooms. The hope is that students around the world will receive the amplified benefits of stress reduction and less loneliness, anxiety, and depression with safe touch added to their yoga practice. For this reason, safe touch must start making its way into trauma-informed yoga classes too. The research[1] proves that safe touch is even more beneficial for individuals with clinical disorders. Every benefit discussed in chapter 1 is felt even more so by those healing from trauma. I know this to be true not only through the data and insight from experts, but also from personal experience. At the time of this writing, touch currently isn't a popular application in trauma-informed yoga, but it needs to be.

I hope to convince you, the trauma-informed yoga instructor, why you should offer safe touch in trauma-focused classes and why RBM is the approach for doing this. Based on my experience as both a yoga student with PTSD and a trauma informed yoga instructor, I'll offer suggestions for how RBM can be adapted for this setting. Modifying RBM is simple because I've designed RBM to be conscious of and sensitive to trauma. However, when working with severe cases of trauma, you must consider disembodiment and its effect on personal agency, and I will suggest how you can adapt RBM in light of such circumstances. My hope is to equip you with both the reasoning and the guidance to start bringing energetically and anatomically safe assists into the trauma-informed yoga classroom, because this setting may very well be where students need it most.

While RBM is informed by trauma sensitivity, it is not a treatment for trauma. It is a tool that may be used by qualified trauma-informed yoga instructors as an adjunct to their work—not as a substitute for clinical care.

Why the Rubber Band Method® Has a Place in the Trauma-Informed Setting

Dr. Bessel Van der Kolk is a leading voice in trauma and trauma healing. In his deeply moving and informative book *The Body Keeps the Score*,[2] he points out how important it is to reconnect with one's body to heal, and he explains that touch is one simple, fundamental way in which someone who has experienced trauma can do that. He notes that

> the most natural way that we humans calm down our distress is by being touched. . . . Touch, the most elementary tool that we have to calm down, is proscribed [denounced, forbidden, avoided] from most therapeutic practices. Yet you can't fully recover if you don't feel safe in your skin. Therefore, I encourage all my patients to engage in some sort of bodywork.

I have had countless real-world experiences teach me, irrefutably, that safe touch is beneficial for people who have experienced trauma. I've had students share with me their experiences of having been assaulted and how helpful it was for them to be in my classroom, where they felt safe to be touched again. This safe touch in the yoga setting offers a corrective experience regarding something that is fundamental to human relationships. Ask yourself how important it might be for someone to relearn that touch is not only okay but can also feel good again. I'd like to share two other personal stories that help to highlight the impact safe yoga assists can have on students with trauma.

I was practicing yoga for several years before and throughout my long journey to overcome complex PTSD. I did the asana, the pranayama, meditation, and the like, but I still suffered unimaginable psychosomatic. One of my symptoms was always feeling like I was suffocating; I never felt like I could take a breath. Eventually, I went to an ear, nose, and throat (ENT) doctor to see whether I had a growth that was blocking my airway. After putting a scope down my throat (my psychosomatic pain included so many scopes!), the doctor proclaimed to me, "Oh, you're fine; you're just breathing backward!" Wait, what? What does that mean?

I was in such a perpetual state of anxiety that instead of opening my airway when I inhaled, I contracted or closed it. It was like every inhale was a gasp. The ENT office didn't offer any physical therapy or help in learning *how* to open my airway when I inhaled; I was left to my own body awareness. I suppose it's such a basic function for our bodies that the health care providers just assumed I'd figure it out. However, I was very disembodied (more on this in a bit) at the time, and learning how to correct this felt nearly impossible for me.

Trauma-informed yoga wasn't mainstream at the time, so I was devotedly attending public yoga classes to help myself heal. Breath is at the heart of yoga, so naturally, I brought the challenge to learn how to breathe to my mat. I had a very intuitive and compassionate yoga instructor whom I practiced with regularly. One evening after some time working on this, I was in her class, still working hard to open my throat on the inhale. I imagine my efforts must have been heard across the studio. Either way, she noticed something going on with me, and she chose to use touch to help.

She would always give us a long savasana and turn off the lights. In this fateful savasana, she came over to me and placed her pinched thumb, index finger, and middle finger on my sternum or breastbone as a nyasa (touching a place on your body to focus awareness). Quietly, so that only I could hear, she said, "Breathe into my fingers." I tried and tried to breathe into her fingers; with each ragged attempt, I only steeled myself further. I'm not sure how long she held the nyasa, but eventually, my throat just opened, and I took the first full, throat-and-chest-expanding breath I had possibly ever taken. Of course, it opened a floodgate, and I remained crying in corpse pose well past the end of class. That was the most powerful healing moment in my life and nothing short of a miracle for me—not just in allowing my brain and body to reconnect on how to breathe but also because of the mental and emotional pain I was able to let go of immediately afterward.

A few years after this experience, I started working for the Art of Yoga Project (AYP), a nonprofit organization that brings yoga and art to incarcerated juveniles. As an instructor for this organization, I had to complete a rigorous and comprehensive trauma-informed training program before AYP permitted me to work with the youths. I remember feeling nervous about teaching my first few classes because, statistically, all the participants had histories of chronic trauma and came from marginalized communities.

Meeting the youths was both intimidating and humbling; I kept having to remind myself that they were just kids. Many of the youths were covered from head to toe in tattoos, including their faces. I recall a couple of girls' faces tattooed with their traffickers' insignias. I also remember my shock when referencing the ocean and *all the youths* saying that they'd never seen the ocean before, although their homes were only a short drive from it. They were all just kids, but each was living a challenging life in countless ways beyond the sentences they were serving.

It was refreshing, as someone with PTSD who had found touch to be so helpful, to be part of an organization that advocates for touch in this setting too. Statistically, all the youths had experienced trauma; most had been members of gangs, and many had been victims of human trafficking. For these reasons, our training included being sensitive to how we taught and touched the students and being conscious of what might be triggering for them. Generally, we were mindful, respectful, and caring, and we always aimed to maintain the girls' personal agency.

We offered assists that were considerate and consensual, and assists became the thing the youths requested most! I would often see a face pop up from child's pose and hear, "Me, me, me! Me next!" Because of the chronic trauma these youths had faced, they would sometimes act out or be difficult to teach. But, over time, the safe assists seemed to soften their defensive exteriors and create space for real connection. The bulk of my memories now are of friendliness and even some smiles and laughter. I remember times when the kids were just getting to be kids. It was through safe touch that walls came down between us and real work could get done among the group.

Personal Agency and Consent

When it comes to offering safe touch in a yoga classroom, the instructor must create and maintain personal agency for each student. Let your mantra forever be *agency, agency, agency*! This is the most critical factor I hope you take from this section and this entire methodology: Receiving touch must be your students' choice, and you must give them the ability to welcome or decline being touched every single time, without ever treating them differently because of their decision. This tenet becomes doubly important in a trauma setting because touch is harmful if the student doesn't feel that it's consensual; the student with trauma must feel they are welcoming touch for it to be safe and beneficial.

As we know, touch isn't often offered in the trauma setting. What most teachers don't realize is that by not offering assists, they are taking away the students' agency. By choosing *not* to offer touch, a teacher is assuming their students don't want to be touched and thus deciding for them. True personal agency is having the power to decide and communicate authority and boundaries for oneself; it's advocating for one's personal wants and needs. It's being given the choice and offered the space to answer. Thus, offering assists and letting the student decide if they wish to receive them is one way to foster agency in the trauma-informed yoga classroom.

For some individuals, their life experience has created a sense of their agency being taken away. When one does not feel like they have power and authority over oneself and one's body, it can lead to disassociation or disembodiment. Those who have experienced being disembodied often describe it as feeling like you are numb—numb to the sensations of your body, your feelings, yourself. It's almost like you've stepped outside of your body and are existing somewhere adjacent to yourself. It's hard to practice personal agency when you feel so disconnected from "you." As an instructor to individuals experiencing disembodiment, when you cultivate an atmosphere in which you create, demonstrate, practice, and uphold agency, you create an opportunity for these individuals to gradually become more and more embodied.

When a trauma-informed yoga teacher offers to provide RBM assists, encourages each student to accept or decline each assist, and always respects the student's choice, that teacher is fostering and upholding personal agency. When the instructor requests permission to provide assists, the student gets to cultivate embodiment by exercising personal choice and cultivating a sense of self through choice. If the student elects to receive assists, the assists can help cultivate embodiment through the heightened kinesthetic feedback of grounding, stretch, or ease; these are the cues that help to hone proprioception, which is exactly what the RBM assists aim to cultivate. Touch helps the disembodied student better attune to their body by amplifying kinesthetic cues the student might otherwise have been numb to and can now focus on and sense (just like a nyasa).

For students who may be too disembodied to make an informed decision, they need to know precisely what they are saying yes or no to. In a public classroom, we can generally request permission for all assists and all adjustments (touch in general) at the start of class, and that will suffice for the duration of class. However, when doing focused trauma work where disembodiment may be present, it's important to receive permission for each individual assist or adjustment. This requirement makes it ideal to co-teach with another instructor so that you can demonstrate the assists for your students, giving them the chance to see what they are participating in. For example, if you plan to teach downward dog front press, supine twist spinal lengthening, and corpse-pose neck traction, you would demonstrate these at the start of class so that the students know what they're saying yes or no to. After demonstrating the assists that you will provide in class, you'd individually ask the student if they'd like to receive each specific assist (referring to it by name) later in the class.

In my experience teaching in a trauma-informed setting, these classes are not overly formulaic or formal, so you have some freedom in how you introduce assists. For example, you could pause and demonstrate each assist with your co-instructor right before offering it rather than demonstrating all assists at the beginning of class. As another option, if you've been teaching several classes to the group and the students are familiar with the assists and their names, you could simply ask by providing the assist name and a short description without demonstration—for example, "Would you like to receive downward dog front press with an assist to your lower back and hips?" However you choose to inform your students of *how* you will touch them, find a way to ensure the students know what they are consenting to.

In the trauma setting, it's still important to request permission in a discreet and tactful way. Assist cards or coins are a great option for this. However, in my experience with trauma-focused work, individuals often respect one another's choice not to participate, and there's less stigma around participation than in the public class setting. Read your room, always uphold agency, and do your best to support private autonomy.

Putting this all together, how might a teacher offer RBM assists in a trauma-informed yoga classroom and receive consent from students who may be feeling disembodied and still cultivate personal agency? At the start of class, give each student an assist coin or card that has *consent* on one side and *decline* on the other side. Inform them of how they can turn the coin or card up or down at any point throughout the class to communicate their choice.

At the beginning of class, demonstrate the two or three assists you intend to offer the class that day and call them by name—for example, downward dog front press, supine twist spinal lengthening, and corpse-pose neck traction. Reiterate how students should use the coin or card, and ask students to turn it to one side to start. At this point, they are generally saying yes or no to touch in general. As the class proceeds, you'll ask permission for each assist by name and invite them to change their card or coin if they so choose for that particular assist. I invite you to reassure the students that at any point, if they wish for an assist to stop or if they change their minds, they can always shake their head no or tell you, "No, thanks." That being said, if the coin or card says no, the choice is respected, and further requests to provide touch won't be made to the student unless they flip the coin or card back over to the side granting consent.

Permission granting is based on informing the student of each assist and receiving consent from each person you offer the assist to. I encourage you to make this process simple and accessible, putting it into practice in your own way as a trained trauma-informed yoga instructor.

A few final thoughts on consent are in order. If you have a rapport with your individual students and the whole group, that is wonderful. Building trust is important to a beneficial student–teacher relationship. However, sometimes rapport can lead you to make assumptions and cut corners. In the trauma-informed yoga setting, even if you have received permission to assist a student countless times, still ask permission every time anyway. Never act based on what you assume the student wants; that is taking away the student's agency, which is the exact opposite of the atmosphere we are aiming to foster. The most unlikely thing can trigger trauma, and you don't know what your student might be feeling from practice to practice. Always ask permission to perform assists, and only provide them when students have granted explicit permission.

Please never take a student's decline of an assist personally. RBM maintains that each student has agency over their body and must feel welcome to invite or decline touch. One way a teacher can take it personally in this setting is by ceasing to offer the invitation to give assists after receiving constant declines to be touched. In the past, I have had students with PTSD for whom it took months before they welcomed touch, but eventually, they did. There was no guarantee of that, but had I stopped offering, they would have never been able to explore the experience of safe touch through RBM yoga assists.

Rubber Band Method® Modifications for Trauma

Every aspect of the RBM approach to assisting applies in the trauma setting; Avoid offering assists when students are in misaligned poses, all the techniques and stances remain the same, as do the tenets of touch. The caveats include how permission is requested (as covered in the previous section), how many assists you offer in general throughout class, and which assists you offer.

In any trauma-focused class, the goal is to reduce stimuli. The healing a participant experiences from trauma-informed yoga results from the settling of the nervous system, whether it be from the poses, breath work, meditation, mantras, or assists. Someone with PTSD has a chronically stimulated nervous system, so the setting aims to reduce rather than increase the feeling of stimulation. For this reason, keep it simple. The assists outlined in this volume are ideal for working with trauma. Advanced assists can be more stimulating for both the student and the teacher and should be avoided in this setting.

Offering several assists can also be too stimulating. I suggest limiting hands-on work to two or three different assists throughout the class. Along with offering fewer assists, I also recommend holding the assists for longer than you would in a public class. This allows the student to better absorb and be present for the kinesthetic cues they're receiving. The methodology already emphasizes entering and exiting poses slowly, but a slower, more prolonged assist can also help to reinforce stillness and calm. You can think of this as four or five breaths in an assist versus one to three breaths.

As mentioned, if a student has a specific physical injury, we wouldn't offer an assist that targets that area. When it comes to mental and emotional injuries, such as trauma, we want to avoid assists that could be retraumatizing or triggering. Assists that can be triggering to someone who has experienced trauma from assault would include chest, shoulder, and hip presses. Furthermore, as a general rule, avoid offering assists that involve placing your hands on the thighs and glutes, which includes all the assists covered in chapter 9, Thigh and Hip. Note that demonstrating the assist is especially key if you plan to place your hand on the student's sacrum or anywhere near their hips (e.g., supine twist). In my experience, the lower back region is totally fine, but remember to read your room and request consent.

Here's a list of the assists in this book that are generally safe to include in trauma-informed yoga classes:

- Corpse-pose arch palpation
- Corpse-pose leg lift
- Locust-pose foot anchor (Note: This could be offered in the cobra variation if locust is too stimulating.)
- Child's pose sacral press
- Child's pose spinal lengthening
- Downward dog front press
- Supine twist spinal lengthening
- Deer-pose spinal lengthening
- Corpse-pose neck traction

With time, students may welcome all assists in this book. However, it's a safe place to start to limit the assists you offer to those in the previous list or fewer, depending on your unique group focus.

At the close of this chapter, I hope you now have a better under-standing of how beneficial safe touch can be for the student healing from trauma. RBM is fundamentally energetically and anatomically safe. With minor modifications, RBM can be an effective technique to complement a trauma-informed yoga program and bring safe touch into the classroom. We're living in a world where most of us are relatively touch-starved, and this is often especially applicable to individuals with trauma. However, touch is vital to the health and well-being of all humans, including those who have experienced trauma. In myriad ways, beyond what's shared in this book, safe touch was my salvation and precisely why I feel called to help bring RBM into the trauma-fo-cused setting. Healing is possible, and RBM can help.

6
PUTTING IT ALL TOGETHER

RUBBER BAND
METHOD® IN ACTION

Now that we've learned about every aspect of the Rubber Band Method®
(RBM), let's put it all together into a step-by-step guide to bring RBM into
the classroom. There are three portions of class to consider when offering
RBM assists. The first is tactfully requesting permission and discreetly
receiving consent at the beginning of class. The second is selecting the
appropriate student for the assist you wish to give and implementing the
incremental steps to follow to provide the assist during the class. The
third is asking permission *again* if you'd like to incorporate essential
oils in your savasana assists near the end of class.

BEFORE PROVIDING ASSISTS

Before the class has begun or at the very beginning of the class, create
a tactful way to ask permission to provide touch and a discreet way
for students to answer. A tactful approach means that it's easy for the
student to answer in whatever pose they're in. If the students are in
savasana at the start of class, for example, simply ask them to place
a hand on the belly to signal an answer. If the students are in child's
pose, ask them for two thumbs-ups. You can create a discreet way
for students to provide their answers by ensuring that students' eyes
are fully or partially closed, they're in a prone or face-down position,
or they need very little movement to signal their response.

When requesting permission, you ask students to opt out or demonstrate in some way that they do not wish to be touched. The students
who have not indicated their choice to opt out are the students you
can provide assists to throughout the class.

Employing assist coins or cards is another tactful and discreet
method.

PROVIDING AN ASSIST

- Select a student who appears comfortable; is holding a safely,
  aligned pose that's suitable to assist; and has no known applicable injury or pain to the region affected by the assist.
- Visually identify the anchor and stretch placements, as well as
  the lines of the pose. Ensure that the handholds are accessible
  and that there are no obstructions around the student that might
  limit your ability to find a stable stance.

- Find your stance fully in the student's space. Before placing your hands on the student, be sure you feel comfortable and are close enough to the student to avoid reaching. If you notice that you need to adjust your stance after placing your hands on the student, do so before applying pressure and starting the assist.

- If providing both anchor and stretch placements, apply the anchor first. Determine what tool you're using to place the anchor. Make sure you have a good handhold before applying pressure to the anchor; if you need to change your hand placement, do so. Once you have applied the anchor pressure, maintain pressure throughout the assist; you apply the anchor first and release it last.

- Determine what tool you're using to place the stretch. Apply the stretch placement by first sinking into the student's tissues with the preferred tool and then ensuring you have a good handhold. If your hand placement feels off in any way, change the placement and ensure it feels secure before applying directional pressure.

- With a secure handhold with the stretch tool, direct your hand along the lines of the pose. Ensure the directional pressure you apply follows the alignment of the shape, mimics the action, or accentuates the lines of stretch present in the pose.

- Slowly apply pressure with your stretch hand until you feel the tissues become taut and then start to pull back, or resist more stretch. This is the dense edge and is the student's safe boundary of stretch.

- At the boundary of stretch, maintain the anchoring pressure and stretch pressure simultaneously for a few moments or breaths. I don't specifically count my breaths or time the length I hold an assist. Simply hold the assist for a few moments or for however long it feels appropriate and comfortable for you.

- When backing out, maintain the anchor pressure as you slowly release the stretch placement. Once you release the stretch placement, release the pressure in the anchor placement last. If you are only applying one of these tools in the assist, the anchor or the stretch, slowly release pressure in both hands simultaneously.

• Once your hands have released the effort or directional pressure of the assist, keep your hands on your student for a brief moment to ensure that their balance is steady and stable and that their tissues have returned to their natural resting position. Release your hands completely before carefully stepping out of their space.

ENDING CLASS WITH ESSENTIAL OILS

When ending a class with essential oils, introduce them when students have just settled into their final resting pose but before they've dropped deeply into the pose. Tell the students which essential oil (e.g., lavender) you plan to use and which assist you will be giving (e.g., savasana neck traction). Ask your students to indicate whether they wish to decline this assist or wish not to be touched. I recommend avoiding assisting anyone who declines the assist with essential oil to ensure you don't lose track of who opted out.

When walking around the room to offer an assist to students in savasana, whether with essential oils or not, to assist the neck or the feet, rub your hands together near each student you aim to assist to alert them to your presence before touching them.

SUGGESTIONS FOR LEARNING

You will need to recruit some friends and colleagues to help learn the RBM approach to assisting. Most people love the chance to receive yoga assists, so don't hesitate to ask friends who aren't instructors to help you learn. In this section, I'll provide suggestions for practicing the material before you bring it into your classroom or offer it to private clients.

My first suggestion is to work one on one with a friend or colleague. You could explore various assists and get a feel for finding a safe stance, reliably locating the anchor and stretch placements, creating secure handholds, reading tissues, and clarifying the purpose of the assist. Be sure to receive the assists as well if you're working with a colleague. Feeling the assist can help to solidify its purpose and aid in interpreting tissue bounds.

Next, be sure to practice on both anatomical sexes. Bodies are shaped differently. The anatomical male and female pelvises are different from one another. When you offer an assist for downward dog front press, the bones can feel markedly different when assisting an anatomical male versus an anatomical female. This is also true of the femur and pelvis in supine twist.

Additionally, body mass and height present different scenarios for assisting. For example, if someone's body mass is greater, it may be more difficult to find the bony landmarks for the handholds of the anchor and stretch using visual cues, and it may require more depth to get a good handhold. If someone is much taller or shorter than you, you'll need to adapt the assist you use for downward dog accordingly. Height also affects how you adjust your low-lunge stance in supine twist spinal lengthening. Because of these anatomical differences, it is important to practice on as many body types as you can before bringing the assists into your classroom.

When you are ready to bring the assists into the classroom, I suggest starting with one assist at a time. You're already juggling a lot, from holding space and sequencing to theming and possibly music coordination. Hands-on assists require an extra layer of management in the classroom. This can feel daunting when you try to add too much too soon. I've seen my trainees do this, and they resort to winging it, which often compromises both their stance and their technique. This isn't safe for them or their students. So, start small!

I suggest planning one assist at a time into your sequence. Plan the pose and assist a few times throughout your class. For example, maybe you teach sun salutations in your vinyasa class and would like to work on downward dog front press. Make a note in your sequence to teach the sun salutations three times and hold downward dog for five or more breaths so that you don't feel rushed each time you give the assist. If you want to work with child's pose sacral press, make a note in your sequence to build in child's pose between kramas (waves of poses), and have your students hold the pose for five or more breaths. Planning the pose and assist in this manner will ensure you can practice the assist on a few different students.

If building the assists into your teaching feels like too much to juggle at first, consider assisting one of your colleagues' classes. This is how I train teachers in teacher trainings (YTT). After working on the assist together in the training, I invite them into my classroom to walk around the room and solely provide assists. This removes the juggling aspect of simultaneously teaching and allows them to focus solely on assisting. If you use this technique, be sure the teacher leading the class asks permission from their students for you to assist them.

Last but not least, if you feel like you'd like more instruction on how to offer RBM assists, you can always take a continuing education workshop or sign up for an on-demand training on the Rubber Band Method® website. In these trainings, I cover the assists in detail and provide a more multidimensional experience of how to step into your student's space and offer an RBM assist.

The Yamas and Niyamas of Rubber Band Method® Assisting

The yamas and niyamas of the yoga sutras are codes of conduct for any aspirant aiming to walk the path of a yogi. They can be applied to just about anything in life, including how to ethically offer hands-on yoga assists.

The Yamas of RBM Assists

- *Ahimsa (Nonharming).* Have the intention, or sankalpa, to always provide energetically and anatomically safe assists. Do this by asking and receiving permission; understanding the purpose of each assist; having a comfortable, stable stance; and reading your student's tissues and adapting your touch accordingly.
- *Satya (Truthfulness).* Never "fake it till you make it" when offering assists. Be sure to practice the techniques with colleagues and friends before attempting assists with your students in the classroom.
- *Asteya (Nonstealing).* Assists always *assist* the pose and asana practice and should never detract from it physically, mentally, or emotionally. Aim to support your students by knowing the purpose of each assist and not detracting from their practice with hurtful touch.
- *Brahmacharya (Abstinence).* Assists are never, ever sexual or sensual. Always respect your own boundaries and your students' boundaries.

- *Aparigraha (Noncoveting).* Remember that by offering the assist, you aren't trying to push your student into a more advanced variation of the pose. Instead, appreciate exactly where they are by allowing the pose to be as it is when you assist. If the student goes further on their own, with you as an objective supporter, that's okay too.

The Niyamas of RBM Assists

- *Saucha (Cleanliness).* Aim to be a clean, light presence visiting your student's space. Be mindful of your cleanliness and limit any body odors.

- *Santosha (Contentment).* Aim to be content with the assists you offer. You are never obligated to give assists to your students, whether that be individual students or everyone in the room. Assists are 100 percent optional, and you should only provide them to appropriate students with whom you feel comfortable offering the assist. Please be content with that. You don't owe assists to anyone.

- *Tapas (Self-Discipline).* No matter how many times you may have taught the same students, remain disciplined enough to ask permission every time you teach a class, and only offer assists to the individuals who have given their consent. Remember that you are creating a culture in your classroom; by asking for permission, you're upholding personal agency and ensuring that everyone you touch feels safe to be touched.

- *Svadhyaya (Self-Study).* Practice, practice, practice! Learn from your friends and colleagues, and then continue to learn from your students. There are mistakes and growing pains in any new endeavor one aims to learn. Don't let mistakes derail you. Remember your wholesome intention of providing safe touch, learn from your mistakes, apply the lessons, and move on.

- *Ishvara Pranidhana (For the Greater Good or Purpose).* Occasionally, let all the positive feedback you're getting from your students really sink in; remind yourself of all the good you're bringing to your students' practice and lives. You are serving the greater good, which makes a significant contribution to your community and the world at large.

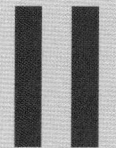
TECHNIQUES

7

RUBBER BAND METHOD® STANCES

High-Squat Stance
Warrior I Stance
Low-Lunge Stance
Low-Squat Stance
Kneeling Stance
Easy-Seat Stance

Many years ago, I had a student who was nearly a foot taller than my height and at least a hundred pounds heavier. He was a tall, muscular man whom I tried to assist using poor body mechanics. I was using my arms to reach opposite points of his body and leaning over him to do so, which loaded my lower back and led to an injury. That moment made me realize that a truly safe assist must be safe for the teacher and the student.

All assists begin with how the teacher holds their body. You can easily injure yourself with poor body mechanics, and you can even compromise your student if your posture is unstable. For this reason, you must always maintain good body mechanics and feel comfortable assisting a student.

Good body mechanics during assists requires the use of the legs to support the arms, maintenance of a straight spine, bones stacked with the shoulders over or behind the wrists, steady balance, comfort within the stance, and only marginal effort for the overall action of the assist. If these elements aren't present in your stance when offering an assist, then you are compromising yourself, the student, and the assist.

Over the years, I have found six stances that meet these criteria for good body mechanics that instructors can use to assist students, whether the student is standing, seated, or lying down:

1. High-squat stance
2. Warrior I stance
3. Low-lunge stance
4. Low-squat stance
5. Kneeling stance
6. Easy-seat stance

All the stances, except for easy seat, are geared toward allowing you to move in and out of multiple assists if you so choose. Usually, easy seat is ideal for one-on-one private clients or in restorative yoga classes, where the holds are for several minutes and you have ample time to make assists.

Almost every teacher I have trained wants to overrecruit their arms when offering an assist. Because it is so common, I'd like to address the use of the arms a bit further. The overrecruitment of the arms likely results from body awareness. We're very attuned to our arms and use them all the time; in everyday life, we don't often recruit our legs to help our arms. However, when you learn to rely on your lower body for strength, your assists are steadier and stronger, and you won't become fatigued as quickly. If you solely use your arms to assist throughout an entire class, you're bound to get fatigued. Recruit your larger, stronger leg muscles to help you stay strong and stable throughout class. The technique section for each stance will teach you how to do this.

Steady balance is also a key component of a strong stance. Balance is critical because Rubber Band Method® (RBM) assists are meant to be helpful and supportive to the student. If you fall on top of your student, that's not helpful. Furthermore, if your lack of balance leads to knocking your student over (yes, it can and has happened!), it can be upsetting and even scary for your student.

If you have sensitive knees and deep flexion or bending is painful for you, you can usually modify the low-squat and kneeling stances with low-lunge stance. Depending on how low to the ground your student is, you may even use easy-seat stance instead. Regardless of your preferred stance or modification, remember that your body comes first. Do not sacrifice your knees or any other part of your body to offer assists. If you feel unsteady, unsure, or uncomfortable, stop the assist and change your stance. If it's not possible to find a stable, supported stance to offer the assist, don't give the assist.

Rubber Band Method® Proper Body Alignment

The legs are recruited to support the strength of the arms.

The spine is straight without loading the lower back.

Bones stack as often as possible—shoulders behind or over the wrists.

Balance is steady and stable.

The stance is comfortable to hold for an extended time.

The action of the assist requires minimal effort.

High-Squat Stance

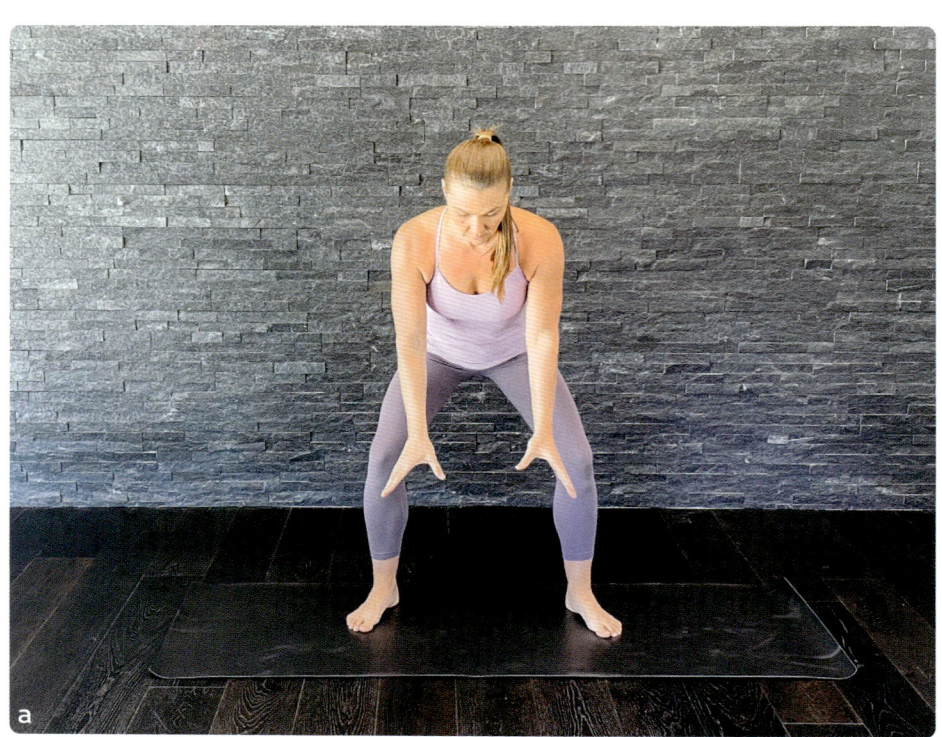

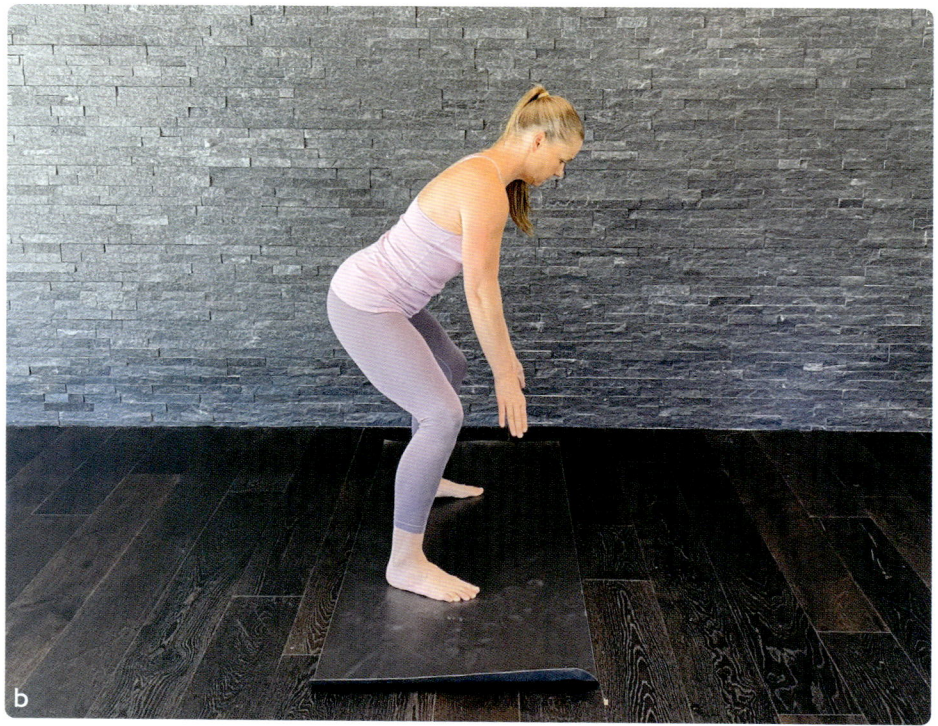

Stance Overview

High-squat stance is one of the most-used stances. In general, it allows you to offer assists from above your student with intentional pressure directed downward. It's a generally accessible stance that makes using the legs easy.

Alignment

High squat is different from goddess or horse pose, although it shares similar roots. In high-squat stance, your feet are set wider than your shoulders, with your hips and knees bent and your feet turned out, as in the yoga pose. However, you are not aiming to feel a stretch of the adductors (inner thigh). In fact, if you feel an adductor stretch, your stance is too wide. In high-squat stance and every other stance, you should never feel a stretch like you're in an asana pose.

The width and outward angle of the feet will be unique to each teacher; find a position in which you feel that you can't be easily knocked over. I sometimes note with trainees that it's the stance you'd take if you were trying to block a goal in soccer or a tackle in football. It's simply a wide stance with the feet slightly turned out that allows you to root into your legs.

Imagine you are in tadasana, or mountain pose, from the waist up. Step your feet out wider than your shoulders, bend your knees, and send your hips back behind you to bring your chest slightly forward. You should stack your ankles under the knees, with your feet turning out as necessary to support bone stacking and knee comfort. Keep your spine straight, and stack your shoulders over your wrists so that when you bend your knees, you can provide downward pressure through the arms.

Using Your Legs

When using high squat, you want to position yourself over your student so that your shoulders are directly above your wrists and your arms are vertical and straight. In this position, you only need to bend into your knees to transfer the strength from the legs into the arms. Generally speaking, directional pressure is downward in this stance.

Troubleshooting

For the safety of your knees, be mindful not to let them cave inward toward your midline. High squat is different from goddess pose, where you attempt to widen your knees as much as possible. If you have taken too wide of a stance, you will see it when your knees begin to cave inward. In this case, narrow your stance.

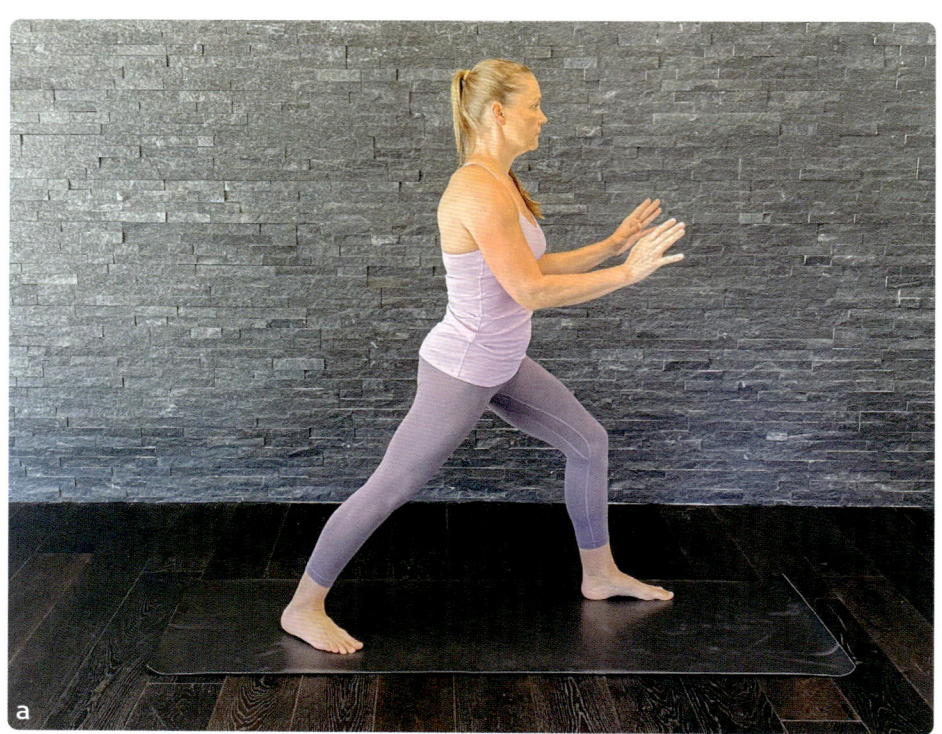

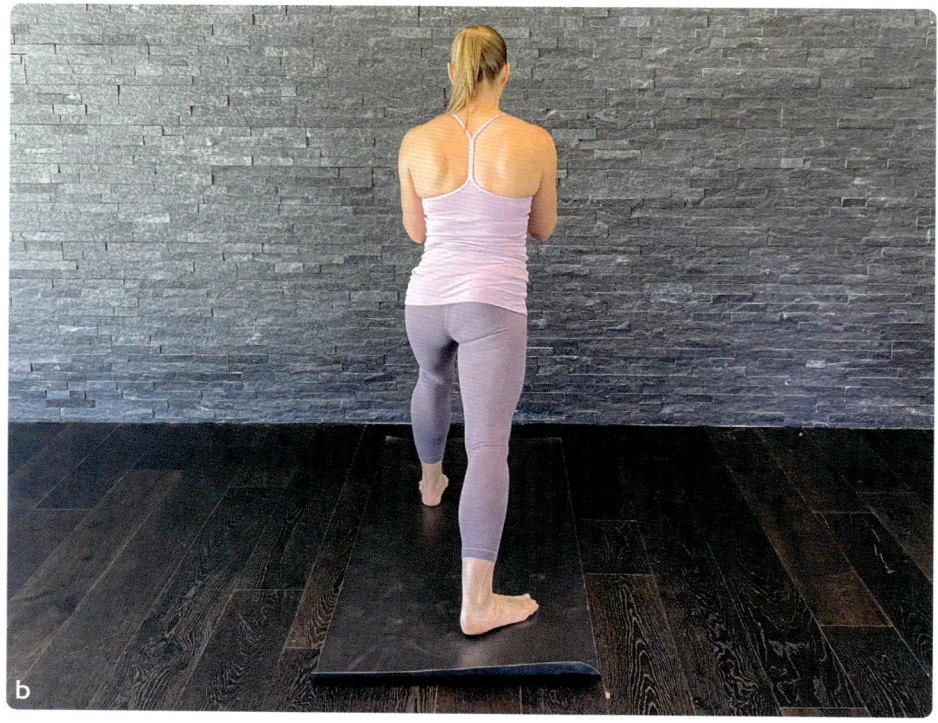

Stance Overview

Instructors generally use warrior I stance to assist postures that are higher off the floor. The directional pressure is often distributed horizontally or parallel to the floor, although not always. Instructors more often use this stance in advanced assists.

Alignment

This warrior I stance is not to be confused with the warrior I pose you would practice on your mat. Many students challenge themselves to go as deep, long, and narrow as possible in warrior I, which is effortful, is not comfortable to hold for a long time, and lacks stability. Warrior I stance is the opposite of the pose you find on your mat, involving a wider and shorter stance.

Do not stand on a tightrope. Your feet should be, at a minimum, shoulder-width apart or wider. Your hips will square toward your student and in the direction you'll be sending the directional pressure of the assist; a wider stance will give you more liberty to do this.

In addition to a wider stance, you want to have a shorter stance. When recruiting the strength of your legs, you'll need to be able to drive off your back leg and bend into your front knee. A long stance won't allow you to do this and will prevent squaring your hips toward your student.

Your elbows will be at your sides, with the upper arms (humeri) held tight to the ribs. Your hands face forward, with the forearms roughly parallel to the floor.

Usually, you will only assist in warrior I stance from your most comfortable side. Do you prefer your left or your right foot forward? Go with the one that's most comfortable for you every time you assist; no need to switch sides in your stance. Not sure? Choose your dominant leg to go backward. You can find it by having someone give you a gentle push from behind; the foot you step forward with first is your dominant leg. This will become your back foot in warrior I stance.

Using Your Legs

When describing how to use your legs, I tell my yoga teacher training (YTT) students, "Find the position you'd take if you had to push a broken-down car off the road." This means that you find a strong stance that helps you feel like you can use the strength of your legs to push. If your stance is too long, it'll be hard to drive through your legs; your back heel will lift when you bend toward your front knee. Consider a shorter stance and a wider footprint that helps you feel as though you can safely bend into your front knee and push off the back heel without it lifting. When you pin your arms to your sides, simply bending into the front knee and driving off the back leg directs the strength of your legs into your hands.

Troubleshooting

Often, students ask, "Why warrior I stance and not a high-lunge position?" The answer is balance. With your back heel lifted, you must manage your balance and your student's balance when you enter their space. Warrior I stance is a modified position that is shorter and wider than a warrior I pose. *This stance aims for stability and strength, not achieving a picture-perfect warrior I.* No one is evaluating your alignment in this shape except you. Do you feel uncomfortable? If so, change your stance by widening or shortening the distance between your feet; make any necessary changes that will help you feel balanced, steady, and able to drive through your legs.

Feel like you're using your arms too much? You're likely standing too far from your student and having to reach. Step farther into their space. Pin your elbows to your sides; the front knee bending forward should be the only movement in the assist.

Low-Lunge Stance

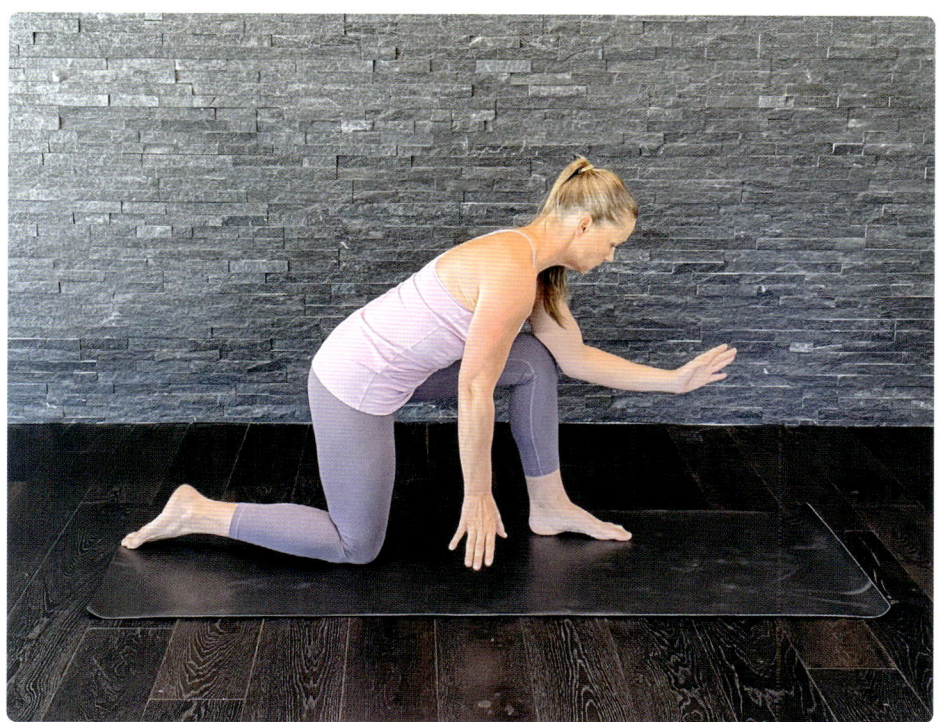

Stance Overview

In addition to high squat, low lunge is one of the most-used stances as you progress through beginner to advanced assists. It allows for steady balance and makes it easy to offer long assists because you use very little arm strength. Usually, you will be assisting seated and supine poses from this stance. Low lunge assists asana poses with two sides, and you will need to be able to assist students with both your right and left foot forward.

Alignment

Nearly every time you offer an assist from low-lunge stance, it's to a pose that has two sides, such as supine twist. Practice both sides: right and left foot forward, with opposite hands acting as the anchor and stretch. The front hand, or the hand on the same side as your front leg, is always the stretch hand. Your back hand, or the hand on the same side as your back leg, is always your anchor hand.

The front thigh is always part of the stance. It applies the directional pressure via the stacking of bones when offering a stretch application; it also offers lower back support when using only an anchor application because it allows you to lean your weight forward and rest your stretch elbow on your thigh.

As with warrior I, let go of this being the low-lunge pose you practice on your mat. Your front foot and back knee may have a shorter or wider distance between them. The point is to find a position that feels comfortable, supportive, and steady.

Low-lunge stance always starts from standing. Observe how your student is positioned on their mat: Are they parallel to their mat, diagonal, or a little of both? Set up your low-lunge stance to mirror your student's body. For example, if I am assisting reclined twist and, from a bird's-eye view, my student's spine is running parallel to the long edges of their mat, I will align my body to theirs along the long edges of the mat. From the same view, if the student is at an angle, with their spine running at a diagonal toward one corner of their mat, I will align my body with theirs and position my low-lunge stance at a diagonal toward the same corner of their mat.

Place your back knee and anchor hand first. Next, place your stretch hand, and then stack the bones from wrist to hip behind it. Your hips will square in the direction in which you will be providing directional pressure; you should be facing and squaring your hips along the lines of the pose.

The distance between the front foot and back knee varies but is often short. You should be able to sink your hips only a little to allow your front knee to bend an inch or so past the ankle and toward the toes. Your back knee is supported by your student's mat or a nearby blanket.

Using Your Legs

You will always stack bones when offering an assist from low-lunge stance. The bone stacking runs from hip to hand, as shown in the example picture of this stance. When the bones stack, you only need to sink your hips slightly, bending into the front knee a little, to distribute the strength of the legs into the hands.

Exercise 1:

- Learn how stacking the bones allows you to sink your hips and bend into your front knee slightly to provide pressure in the assist.

- Find a low-lunge stance with your right foot forward and your back left knee supported by your mat or blanket. With hands at your hips, start to bend into your front knee. Anatomically speaking, your front knee can safely track ahead of your ankle if your personal history doesn't involve knee injuries that make the movement uncomfortable. If it is uncomfortable, back off on the depth of the bend in your front knee. Once you have felt the ability to move the weight of the hips forward and back, add the arms.

- Place your left hand on the floor or block, allowing it to act as the anchor. The shoulder of this anchor hand stacks over the wrist. Then, place your right elbow directly in front of your right kneecap. If viewed from the side, your hip to fingertips would run in a straight line: hip → thigh → kneecap → elbow → forearm → hand. All elements in the line are roughly parallel to the floor. Then, repeat the first step and move the hips forward and back, bending in and out of your front right knee. By placing your elbow in front of your knee, you're stacking your bones from hip to hand, which allows you to sink the hips and apply the directional pressure of the assist. You know you are using your legs if you bend your knee and it pushes your hand forward.

Exercise 2:

• Learn how angling the feet and hips changes the directional pressure of the assist.

- Set the short end of your mat about a foot from a wall. Depending on your height, you may need to modify this distance. Come into a lunge with the toes of your front foot aligned with the short edge of your mat. Square your hips and front foot to the wall. Place your anchor, or back hand, on the ground or a block first. Now, stack your stretch elbow, or front elbow, directly in front of your kneecap, extending your wrist and facing your palm to the wall (like signaling "stop"). Slowly bend into your front knee, sinking your hips. You should be able to close the distance and touch the wall with your stretch hand without needing to reach or remove your elbow from the kneecap.

Let's take this further and demonstrate how placing your back knee and front foot to mirror your student changes the angle of the directional pressure when you sink your hips. Follow the exact steps just described, but place your back knee on the long edge of your mat on the right side. Your front toes now slightly point to the left to line up with the knee. Square your hips toward your front foot. Stack the right elbow at the right kneecap, and extend the wrist to face the palm to the wall. Bend into your front knee. Your palm is no longer touching the wall at the center of your mat; it is a few inches to the left.

Now, try placing your back knee on the other long edge of your mat, on the left side. Adjust the squaring of your hips and the direction you point your front toes. Repeat the exercise. See how your directional pressure has now completely changed? This exercise demonstrates how stacking the bones (thigh and forearm) allows you to use your legs when you sink into your hips. When you change your footprint and angle your body differently, the directional pressure of the assist changes too. For this reason, low-lunge stance must mirror the student's body.

Practice these exercises on both sides with each foot forward and opposite hands acting as the anchor and stretch.

Troubleshooting

I find it easiest to build the bone stacking from hand to hip when offering an assist. Start by mirroring your student's body as you come down beside them in low-lunge stance. Place your anchor and maintain the downward pressure. Next, place your stretch hand, but don't apply any pressure yet. Bend your elbow and inch your front foot to align your kneecap behind your elbow. Once you are aligned from hip to hand, sink the hips and apply pressure in the stretch hand.

If it hurts to drop your back knee, use something to pad your knee. If there is room on the student's yoga mat, I will place my knee on their mat. If there is a blanket prop nearby, whether it belongs to the student I am assisting or another student, I will use it and then return it to its prior position after the assist.

Low-Squat Stance

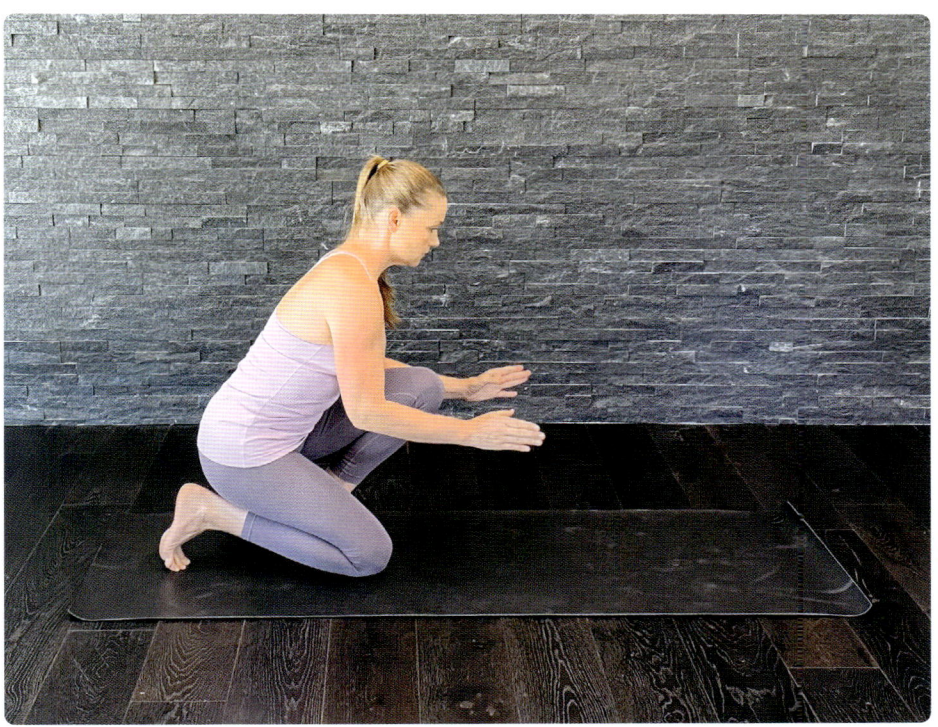

Stance Overview

Low squat is a great option for offering several assists back-to-back. This isn't the pose I use with private clients when more time is available. However, it's great when you have a packed classroom and would like to offer many assists for the same posture. For example, I will often use low squat when providing a chest press in corpse pose in a full classroom.

Low squat is ideal for offering assists close to the floor when the student is either seated or lying down. The benefit of low squat is being able to move up and down easily as you move from student to student without compromising your balance or knees.

With the back knee bent to the floor and the toes tucked, you can move up and down and shift your shoulders forward and back to use the strength of the legs when offering an assist. The directional pressure can be parallel or perpendicular to the floor.

One knee is dropped for all foundational assists taught in this book. With more advanced techniques, both knees are lifted and the knees are utilized as tools for assisting.

Alignment

I think of this position as the one you'd take if you needed something from under the sink. It's simply dropping your back knee to the ground and sitting on your heel with the back toes tucked. Keeping the back toes tucked serves two purposes. First, it allows you to drive off the foot to shift your shoulders forward over your wrists and the student. Second, you can easily press off the toes and quickly return to a standing position.

The back leg is down, with the toes tucked and the knee to the floor. The front leg roots the entire sole of the foot on the floor and the knee bent toward the chest. As always, the spine remains straight in this and all other stances.

Using Your Legs

It doesn't matter which knee you choose to drop to the ground. The knee set to the ground is considered your back knee, and it's the leg you'll drive off to support the strength of the assist. The front foot, the foot fully rooted to the ground, steadies your balance. You can also use this front leg to support the lower back by leaning your chest against the thigh.

When providing the assist, drive off the ball of the back foot to bring your chest forward, and stack your shoulders over your wrists and the student. If you are fully in your student's space, you will not have to reach, and you can easily drive off your back leg to shift your shoulders over your student.

Troubleshooting

The low squat isn't for everyone. If you feel unsteady in your balance or uncomfortable in your hips, knees, or ankles, find a different stance, such as low lunge.

Kneeling Stance

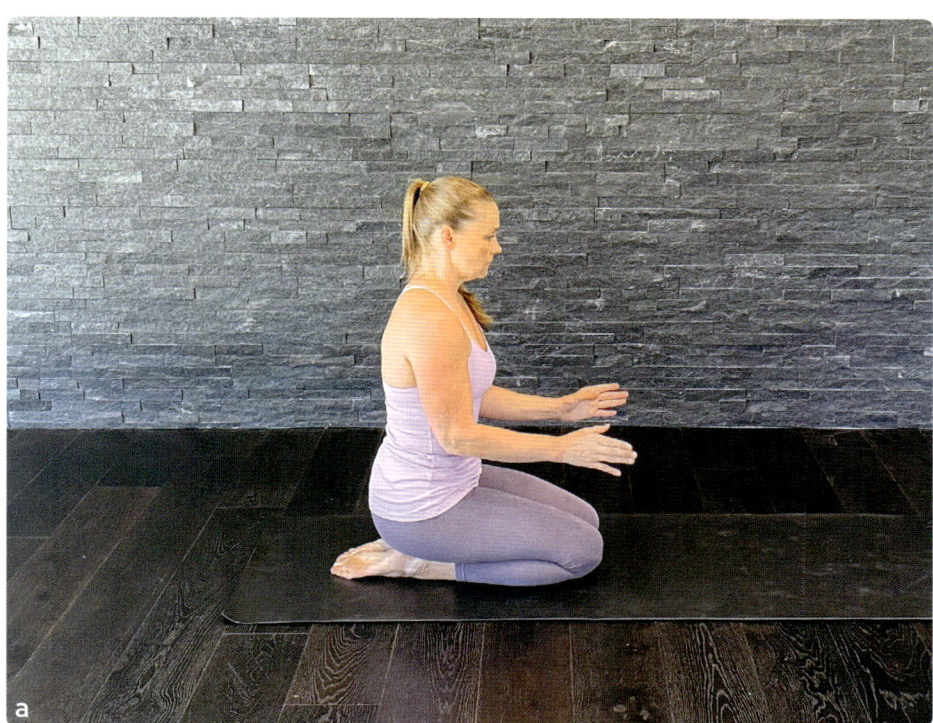

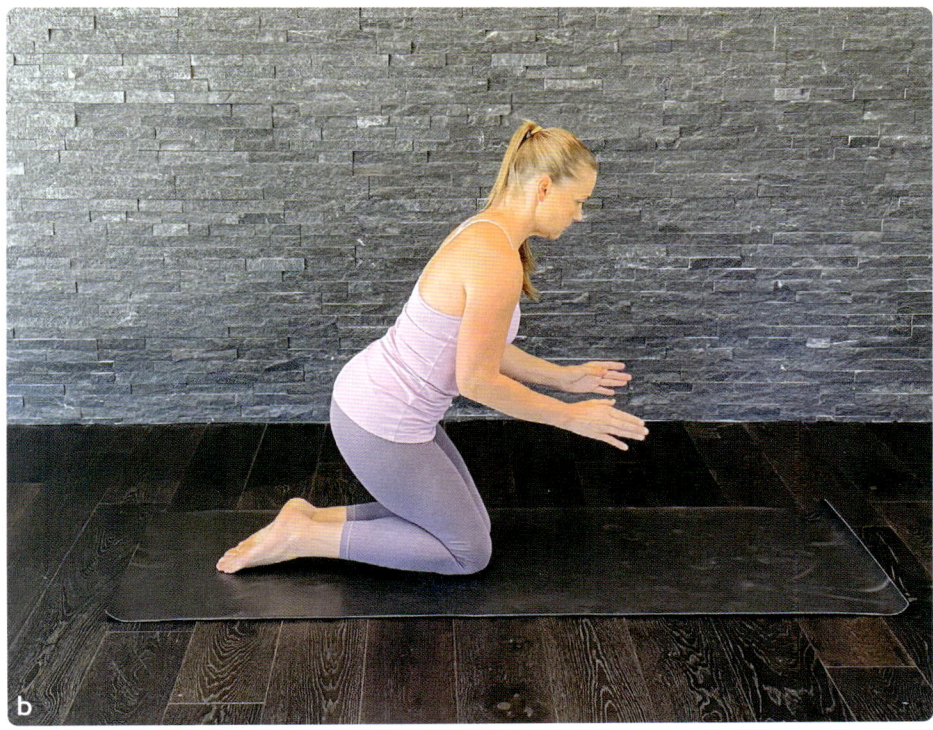

Stance Overview

Kneeling is a great option for offering assists when your student is seated. It's also often effective if your student is in a supine position or lying down. This stance takes a bit more time to come out of, so I don't usually use this pose if I'm aiming to offer several assists to multiple students.

Kneeling stance has two variations: seated on the heels or standing on the knees. Choose which variation is best based on the height of your student in the current pose—for example, based on whether the student is seated, on the floor, or lying on a bolster.

Directional pressure varies with this assist. It can be parallel or perpendicular to the floor.

Alignment

This stance requires placing your knees close to your student. This way, you only need to lean forward slightly to bring your shoulders over your wrists and over your student. Your back should be straight, creating a straight diagonal line from the crown of the head to the tailbone.

The movement of the assist is created by lifting the hips up and forward. By doing this, the chest comes forward, and you can stack your shoulders over your wrists and the student. When the arms are in a locked-out position, it's easy to apply directional pressure downward.

Modify your kneeling stance to accommodate the height of your student. Depending on the height of the student, you can take this stance when seated on the heels with the toes flat or the toes tucked or when standing on the knees. The point is to stack your shoulders over your student while keeping your arms straight.

Using Your Legs

Shifting your chest forward by driving off the toes, the tops of the feet, or the knees in this assist involves the legs. The height of your student will dictate which variation of the legs you choose and how to use the legs in your assist.

If a student is flat on the floor, sitting on your heels with the tops of your feet to the mat will likely suffice. Leaning your chest forward brings your shoulders over your student, and you're driving off the tops of the feet and shins to support the strength of the assist.

If a student is slightly higher, such as a student lying on a bolster, you may stand on your knees and tuck your toes. In this scenario, you're driving off the knees and the tucked toes to bring the chest forward as your hips bend back.

Yet another variation is sitting on the heels but with the toes tucked. In all these variations, the point is to adjust your legs to be able to place your shoulders over your student with straight arms and a straight spine. Driving off the tops of the feet, toes, or knees will bring your shoulders forward.

Troubleshooting

If you find yourself leaning over your student and your back feels loaded, you are reaching and are not close enough to your student. Reposition your knees closer to the student, and then try the assist again. If that doesn't solve the problem, approach the assist from a different stance, such as low squat, where you can lean your chest against your front thigh.

Depending on the sensitivity of your knees, you could sit on the heels, grab a block to place between your ankles to sit on, or stand more on the knees to open the angle of the joint and reduce the bend. If none of these variations is comfortable for you, consider low-lunge or easy-seat stance instead.

Easy-Seat Stance

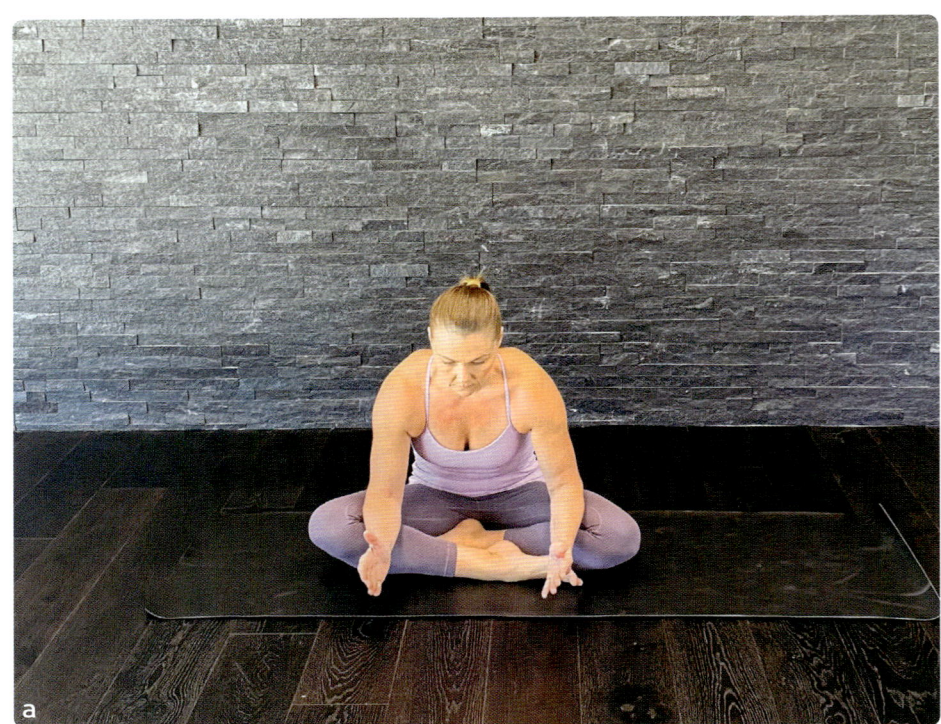

a

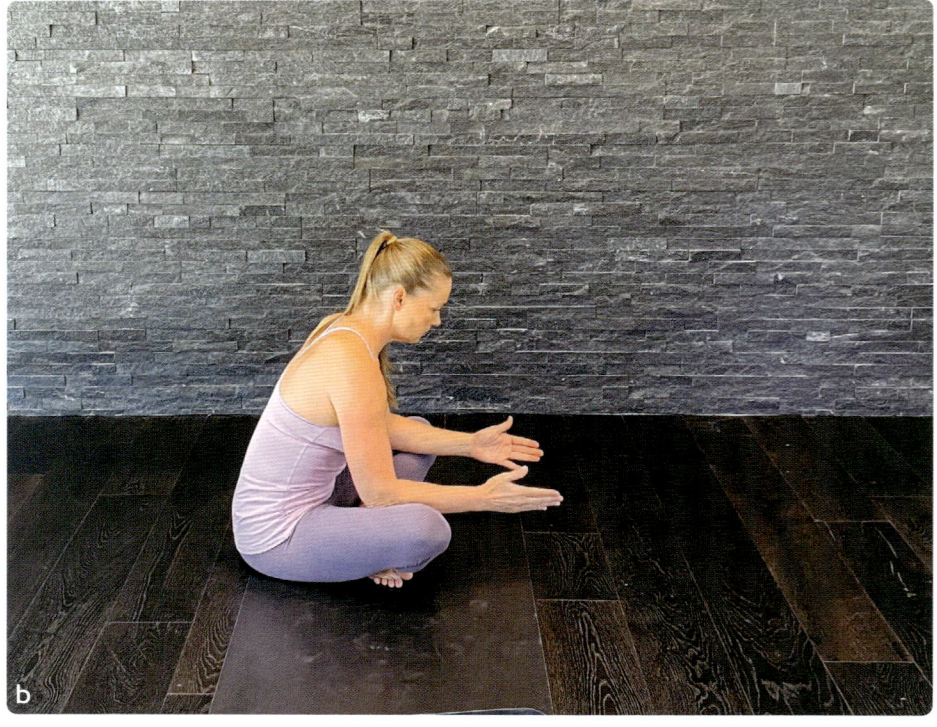

b

Stance Overview

This is the most comfortable stance to provide an assist from. That being said, it takes the most time to come into and out of, so it isn't the best choice if you will be assisting several students. This is a great stance if you have ample time to offer the assist or are working one on one with a client.

This stance is only used when a student is lying in a supine position, such as corpse pose. Directional pressure is limited to the range of motion of the hands because the elbows stay connected to the legs in this stance.

Alignment

This is simply a crossed-leg, seated position. Find any variation that is most comfortable for you and allows you to lean forward and place your elbows on your legs with your back straight. No one is correcting your alignment or evaluating what pose you take. If "crisscross applesauce," or the true variation of sukhasana with the ankles under your shins, is most comfortable for you, take it. If accomplished pose, or siddhasana, with the shins stacked one in front of the other, is more comfortable, then do that. Go with what feels best for you.

Note that you do have to sit rather close to your student to provide an assist from this stance. Avoid reaching from this position because it becomes unstable and can load the lower back. Allow your elbows to rest on your legs. With your elbows resting on the legs, you should be able to contact and assist your student. You can passively lean on the legs and relax a great deal throughout the rest of your body.

Using Your Legs

Use your legs by leaning your elbows on them. This may not seem to support the lower back, but it does. When assisting for a long time and leaning toward your student, your lumbar (lower back) flattens, and your erector muscles (long spinal muscles) are eccentrically holding you up. These muscles get fatigued when you hold this position for a while. Help these muscles and avoid fatigue by using your legs and placing your elbows on them.

It doesn't matter where you place your elbows on your legs. For me, stacking one shin in front of the other is most comfortable, so my elbows land on my calves. Depending on which variation of the crossed-leg seat you choose to take, your elbows may rest on your knees or lower thighs. It doesn't matter where they fall; just be sure that your elbows are resting somewhere on the legs.

Troubleshooting

Ensure that your easy seat is comfortable and that tight hamstrings are not pulling on your lower back. Have a prop handy for under your seat if your legs are not supporting you and are, instead, hindering your comfort. With my private clients, I will hold assists for two to three times as long as I would in a public class. I do not like to suffer, so I place a blanket under my hips and support my stance before I even touch my client.

Over the years, I've witnessed trainees aim to take an easy seat by finding a wide-leg seat, such as upavistha konasana. I strongly discourage anyone from doing this when offering an assist. First, it provides no support for the elbows, so there's no way to use the support of the legs for the lower back. Also, when you use this stance to offer an assist to floor poses (e.g., corpse pose), wide-leg seat puts your sensitive areas far too close to the student's head without a barrier between them. Keep in mind the comfort and sensitivities of your students when considering sitting with both legs stretched out wide and a student's head between your legs.

8
FEET

Corpse Pose: Arch Palpation
Corpse Pose: Leg Lift
Locust Pose: Foot Anchor

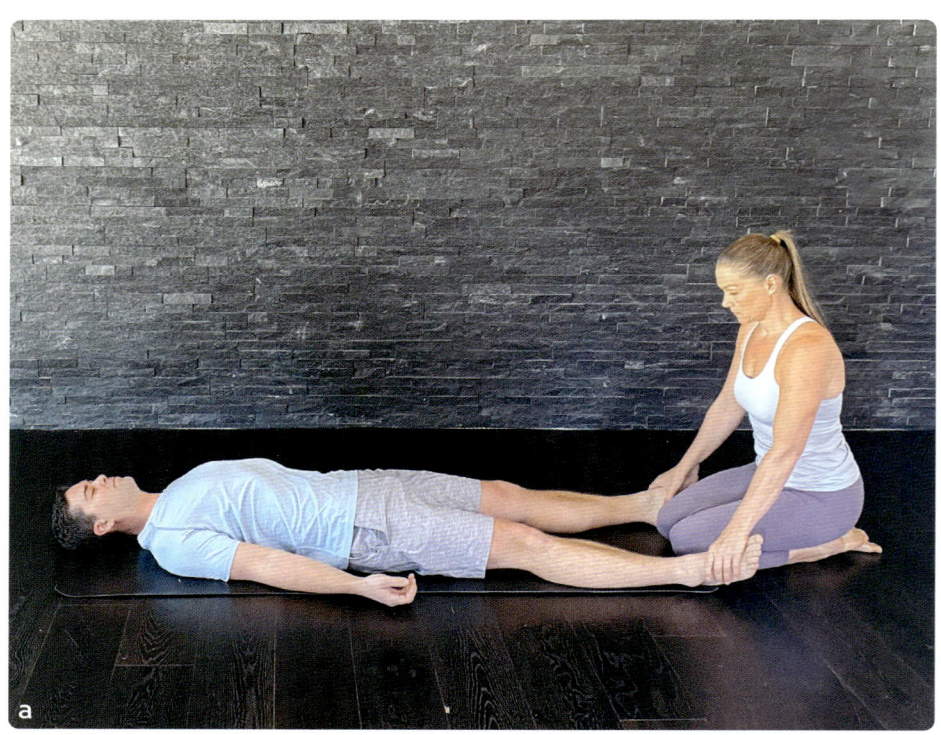

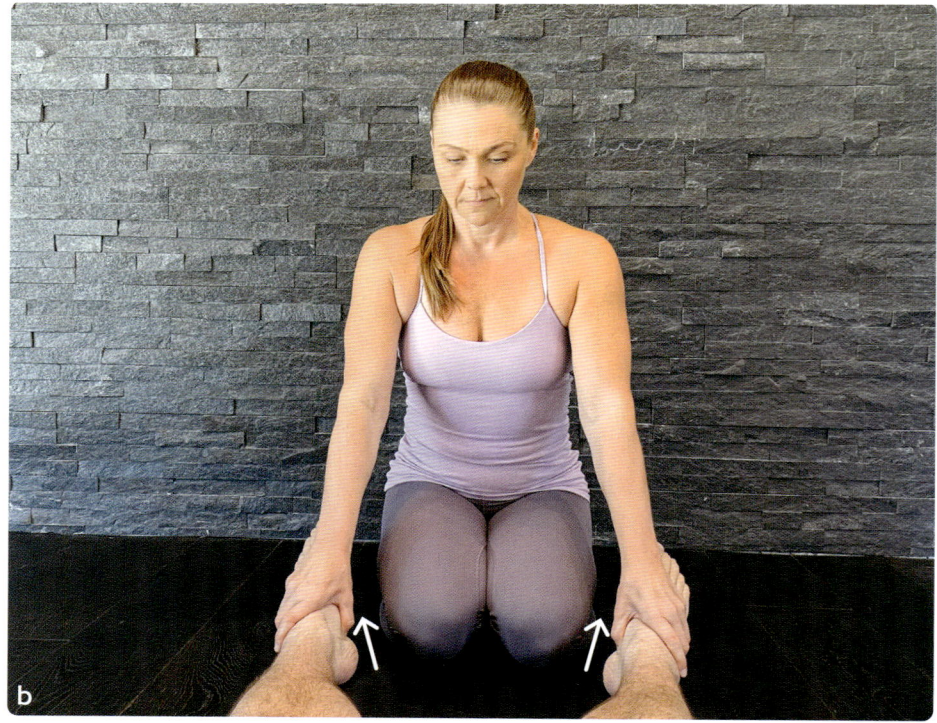

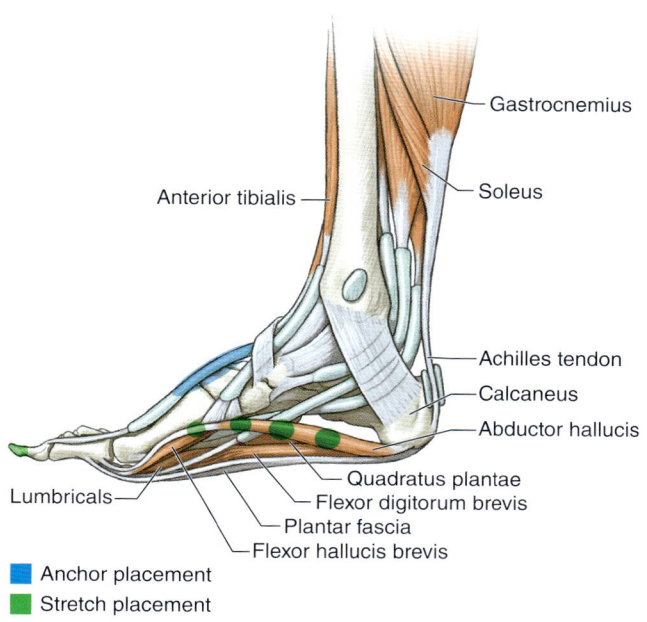

Gastrocnemius

Anterior tibialis

Soleus

Achilles tendon

Calcaneus

Abductor hallucis

Quadratus plantae

Lumbricals

Flexor digitorum brevis

Plantar fascia

Flexor hallucis brevis

■ Anchor placement
■ Stretch placement

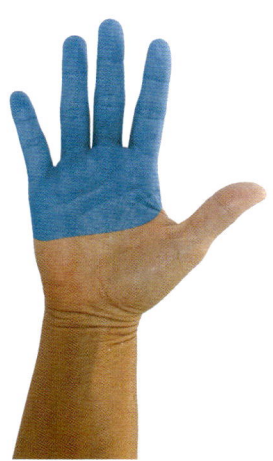

Anchor tool

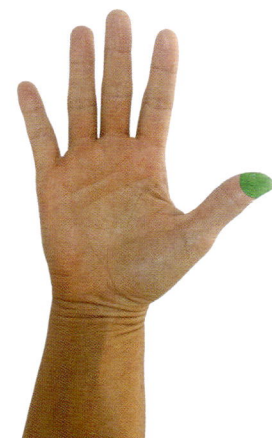

Stretch tool

> ## STUDENT ALIGNMENT
>
> ### Savasana: Corpse Pose
>
> The body is in a supine position.
> The feet are hip-width apart or wider.
> The knees may be supported with a bolster or blanket.
> The arms are open to the sides, with the backs of the hands resting on the mat.
> The head rests on the mat or a prop.

Purpose

Corpse pose, or savasana, is intended to cultivate relaxation and integration of the practice. However, many students struggle to remain present in this pose because their minds wander and drift off. An assist can help the student remain grounded and easeful in the pose. Working with the feet is especially grounding because the feet are the connection points between the body and the earth.

Stance

Kneeling
Alternative: Low Squat

Place both knees between the student's heels. Be close enough to your student that with your arms in a locked-out position, your hands contact their feet. Keep your elbows straight throughout the assist so that you only need to lean your chest forward slightly to distribute weight into the thumbs and, thus, into the assist. This allows you to recruit your legs and entire upper body for the assist.

Anchor Tool

The anchor tool is the palmar surface of your hand and fingers, excluding the thumb. Turn your palms down and point your fingers outward.

Anchor Placement: Dorsal Foot, Top of Foot

Anchor the foot gently in place by wrapping your palm and fingers around the top of the foot. Your fingers will wrap around the pinky edge of the foot to gently hold the foot in place throughout the assist. Be mindful to keep the foot in a neutral position throughout the assist.

Avoid any rotational stress on the student's knee with this anchor placement.

Stretch Tool: Tip of Thumb

The action of this assist is palpation with the thumb. Lock out your thumb to avoid hyperextending the joint. It should look like a straight line from the shoulder to the elbow, through the wrist, and out to the tip of the thumb.

Stretch Placement: Medial Arch

Apply the stretch by pushing your thumb into the soft tissues of the arch of the foot. Each palpation of the thumb serves to gently stretch the myofascia of the medial arch.

Follow the Lines

The lines you are following are along the medial arch. To find the medial arch before offering this assist to a student, stand and palpate the inner arch of your own foot. The portion that is exposed when you are standing is the portion you will palpate on your student.

Palpate from the front of the heel to the big toe. Look for soft tissue rather than bone to press into. Begin at a soft portion of the arch closest to the heel. Press every half inch or so up the length of the arch. You can end on the arch at the base of the big toe or the inner edge of the big toe.

Myofascial Region

This assist compresses the myofascia of the medial (inner) arch of the foot and plantar fascia, mostly the abductor hallucis and flexor hallucis brevis muscles (*hallucis* means "big toe").

General Precautions

Be careful not to hyperextend your thumb. Keep your thumb straight from the wrist to the tip of the thumb to avoid injury to your hand. Most people find that this assist feels good regardless of pressure, so do not concentrate on trying to push very hard. Apply the pressure that feels good for you without strain or much effort.

Common Misalignments

This assist is generally safe for all students. However, if your student has an ankle or foot injury, avoid providing this assist. If they suffer from plantar fasciitis, there is a chance they might be too sensitive for palpation. However, this isn't always the case, so feel free to ask the student rather than strictly avoiding the assist.

If a student has exaggerated external rotation at the hip, the lateral (pinky) edge of the foot presses to the floor when you palpate. Ensure the foot is fully supported with your hand to minimize unnecessary movement; while the thumb palpates, the rest of the hand stabilizes the foot in a neutral position. It is important to hold the foot in place when palpating to prevent any rotational stress at the knee.

Troubleshooting

Remember to use your legs in this assist. You do this by locking out the arms from the shoulder to the thumb and using your legs to rock your chest forward.

Many people are ticklish or sensitive on their feet. Be open to asking if someone wants their feet touched even after receiving permission to provide assists. For example, similar to how you ask permission at the start of class, as soon as students have settled into savasana, ask the room if anyone would like to decline a foot assist.

Never alternate between assists where you touch the feet first and then touch the head. Most people will not appreciate having hands placed on their heads or hands after the teacher has touched another student's feet. Instead, stick with giving foot assists throughout savasana should you decide to offer this assist in a public classroom.

If you are weaving work involving the feet into your sequence, it's a good idea to have hand sanitizer at your mat. After working with feet, if you're going to touch other parts of your students' bodies, give your hands a spritz first.

PUTTING IT ALL TOGETHER

- Be sure the student has space between their feet for you to find a kneeling stance between their ankles.
- If need be, gently clasp the outside of the ankles and part their feet wide enough to find a kneeling stance between the feet. Your knees are aligned inside the student's ankles.
- Place your hands on the tops of the student's feet, with your thumbs facing each other and pointed toward the arch of each foot.
- With your arms straight, subtly lift your hips to rock your chest forward, and then press your thumbs into the soft portion of the arch just ahead of the heel.
- Think of palpating the side of the foot rather than the sole of the foot.
- Using a palpating movement, begin to lean forward, and then press and hold for a moment. Rock your chest back as you release pressure.
- While palpating, move the thumb a half inch or so at a time until you have palpated the length of the arch. Make your way up the arch of the foot toward the big toe.
- Complete the assist by pausing and pressing your thumbs into the soft spot on the inside tip of the big toes.

Corpse Pose: Leg Lift

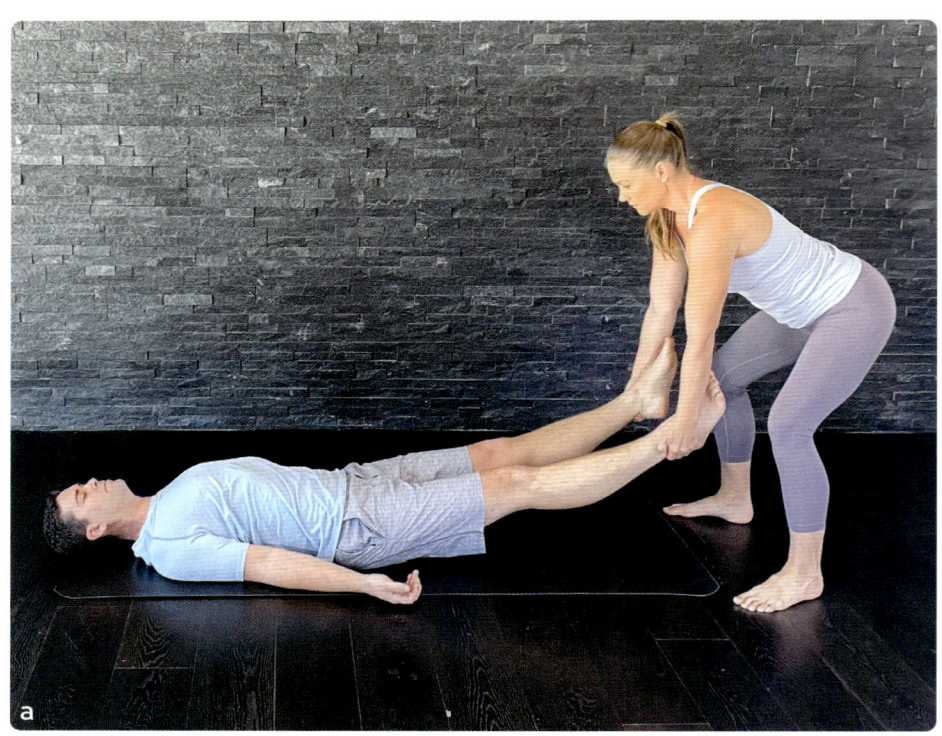

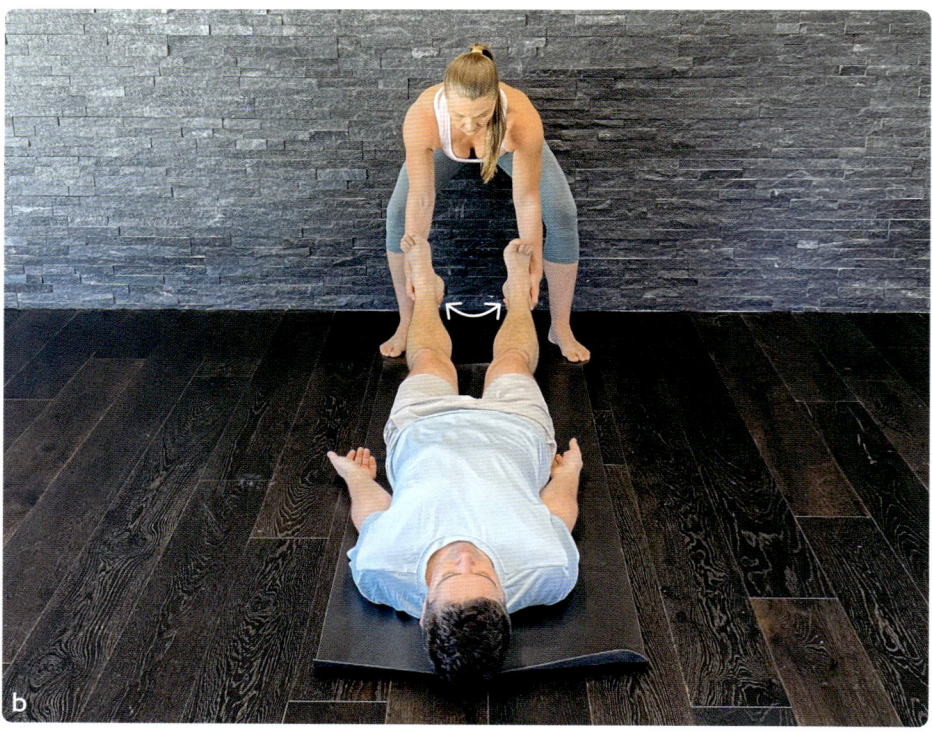

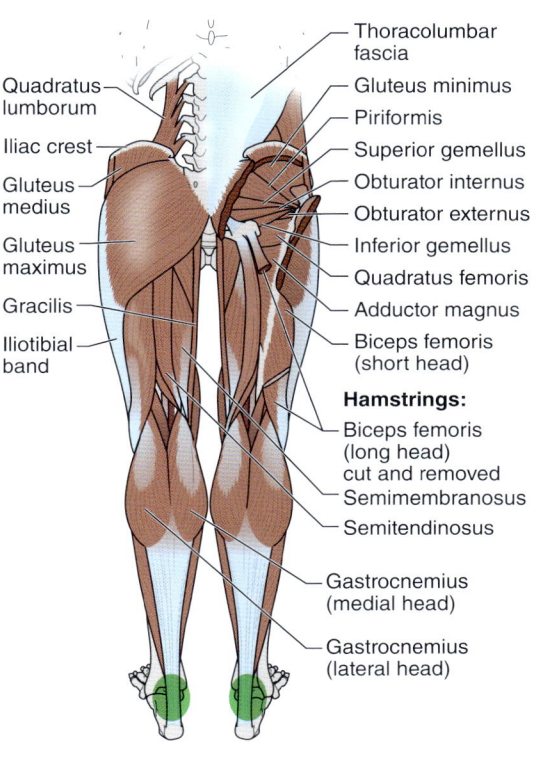

Quadratus lumborum

Iliac crest

Gluteus medius

Gluteus maximus

Gracilis

Iliotibial band

Thoracolumbar fascia

Gluteus minimus

Piriformis

Superior gemellus

Obturator internus

Obturator externus

Inferior gemellus

Quadratus femoris

Adductor magnus

Biceps femoris (short head)

Hamstrings:

Biceps femoris (long head) cut and removed

Semimembranosus

Semitendinosus

Gastrocnemius (medial head)

Gastrocnemius (lateral head)

■ Stretch placement   **Posterior**

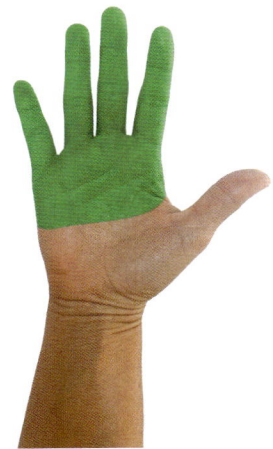

Stretch tool

STUDENT ALIGNMENT

Savasana: Corpse Pose

The body is in a supine position.

The feet are hip-width apart or wider.

The knees are not supported with a prop.

The arms are open to the sides, with the backs of the hands resting on the mat.

The head rests on the mat or a prop.

Purpose

Corpse pose, or savasana, is intended to cultivate relaxation and integration of the practice. However, many students struggle to remain present in this pose because their minds wander and drift off. An assist can help the student remain grounded and easeful in the pose. Lifting and swaying the legs and feet from side to side creates a feeling of weightlessness in the body. Rocking back and forth is a soothing motion that creates greater calm in this final resting pose.

Stance

High Squat

Be sure to step your feet wide enough to keep your back straight as you bend down to pick up the student's feet. Your arms stay straight, with your shoulders over your wrists, throughout the assist. Your feet will not move during the assist; keep them at the same width as you bend over to pick up your student's feet, throughout the top of the lift, and as you return their feet to the floor.

Without moving your feet or bending your elbows, maintain a straight spine throughout the assist. Bend and straighten your knees to use your legs throughout the assist. At first, your knees will bend deeply to lift the student's feet from the floor. At the top of the lift, your knees will straighten somewhat. This is an assist where you can and must recruit your legs rather than using your arms to create the movement in the assist.

Anchor Placement: Provided by the Student

The anchor is created by the weight of the student's torso and pelvis on the mat.

Stretch Tool: Cupping the Fingers

Turn your palms up and curl your fingers to create a cupping shape with both hands. This is the shape you'd make if holding water in your hand. You should be able to softly clasp the student with this tool.

Stretch Placement: Calcaneal (Achilles) Tendon

Coming from the outside of the ankles, clasp your hands around the student's calcaneal (Achilles) tendon. This is the strong tendon found just above (superior to) the heel.

Follow the Lines

This assist isn't aimed at creating a stretch, but we still want to read the lines of stretch to ensure no stretch is created. The lines of stretch run between the heels (stretch placement) and the hips (anchor placement). Be mindful not to lift the feet too high to avoid any tension or stretch along the backs of the legs.

Lift the feet in a circular motion to reduce the pull on the lower back. Instead of lifting directly upward, lift out and up as if each ankle is drawing a half circle. The right ankle lifts out and up to draw the right side of the circle, and the left ankle lifts out and up to draw the left side of the circle. The legs will come together at the top of this imaginary circle.

Using a slow, meditative sway, begin to rock the feet from side to side. Be mindful that you aren't making huge movements and swinging the student's feet wider than their shoulders.

Swing as you lift, but do not exceed a 45-degree angle off the floor. After lifting the legs for a few rocking movements, gently rock the legs back down to the floor. Be mindful that your movement is slow and meditative throughout.

Before letting go of the feet, gently pull the heels toward you to lengthen the posterior chain or back body. This will reduce the curve in the lower back, so after giving the gentle pull, gently push the heels back toward the student to reestablish the lumbar curve in the lower back. After finishing with the gentle pull and push, place the feet lightly on the floor at roughly the same width as you found them.

Myofascial Region

This assist involves the myofascia of the posterior chain: soleus, gastrocnemius, hamstrings, gluteal muscles, quadratus lumborum, and spinal erectors.

General Precautions

This assist is very nurturing and relaxing. However, if you lift the legs too high, it can pull on the hamstrings and lower back. Avoid exceeding 45 degrees or 18 inches (46 cm) of lift from the floor. If someone feels particularly tight without much lift at all, you will feel some resistance from their legs as you lift only slightly. Listen to their body and do not lift any higher.

Keep in mind your stature in comparison to that of your student. If your student is significantly bigger than you, please remember that legs are heavy, and the student's legs might feel especially heavy to lift. I suggest starting out with people who are roughly your size or smaller as you get comfortable with using your legs in this assist.

Common Misalignments

Do not offer this assist to a student who has elected to use a bolster under their knees or has selected a variation of corpse pose such as bound angle or Stonehenge.

Troubleshooting

Never alternate between assists where you touch the feet first and then touch the head. Most people will not appreciate having hands placed on their heads or hands after the teacher has touched another student's feet. Instead, stick with giving foot assists throughout savasana should you decide to offer this assist in a public classroom.

If you are weaving work involving the feet into your sequence, it's a good idea to have hand sanitizer at your mat. After working with feet, if you're going to touch other parts of your students' bodies, give your hands a spritz first.

PUTTING IT ALL TOGETHER

- Assuming high-squat stance, clasp the outside of the student's feet, with your fingers wrapping around the calcaneal (Achilles) tendon just above the heel.

- For a gentle lift, circle the ankles outward, bringing them together at the top of the circle.

- Slowly and gently, begin to rock the legs from side to side, but do not exceed the width of the student's shoulders.

- If you wish, the legs may remain close to the ground as you rock the legs back and forth, or you may lift them up toward 45 degrees, but do not go higher.

- Before you place the feet on the ground, you may wish to lightly pull and push the ankles, offering a light spinal release.

- If you choose to pull and push the feet gently, be sure to end on a push rather than a pull to reset the lower back into a neutral position.

- When placing the feet back onto the mat, leave them relatively close to where you found them (i.e., hip- or shoulder-width apart).

- Be sure the student's feet have returned to their natural resting position before releasing both hands and carefully stepping out of the student's space.

Locust Pose: Foot Anchor

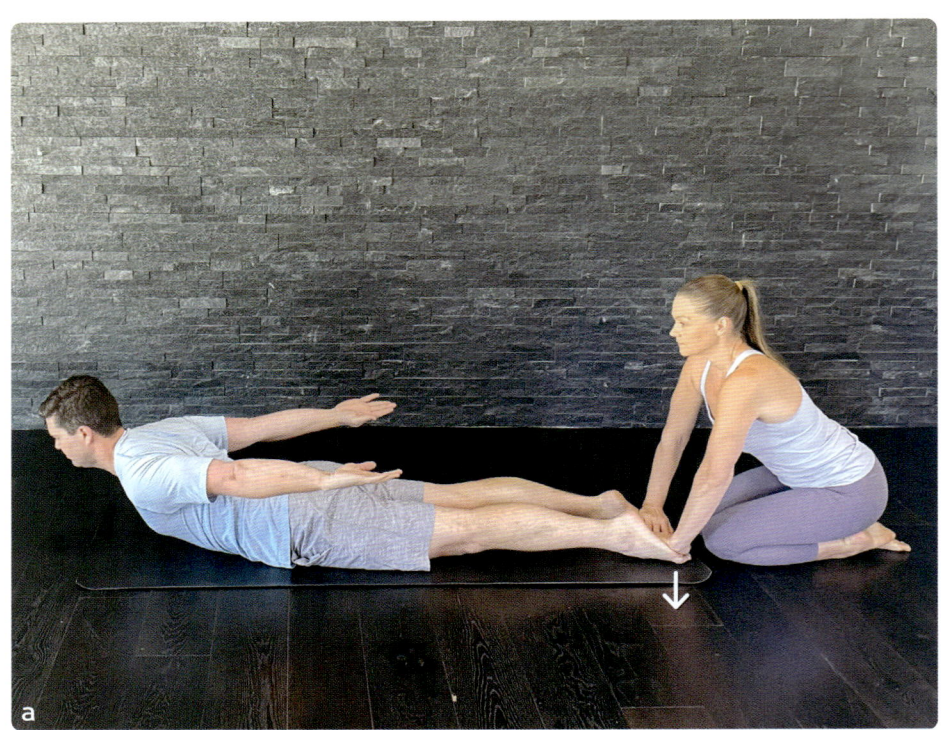

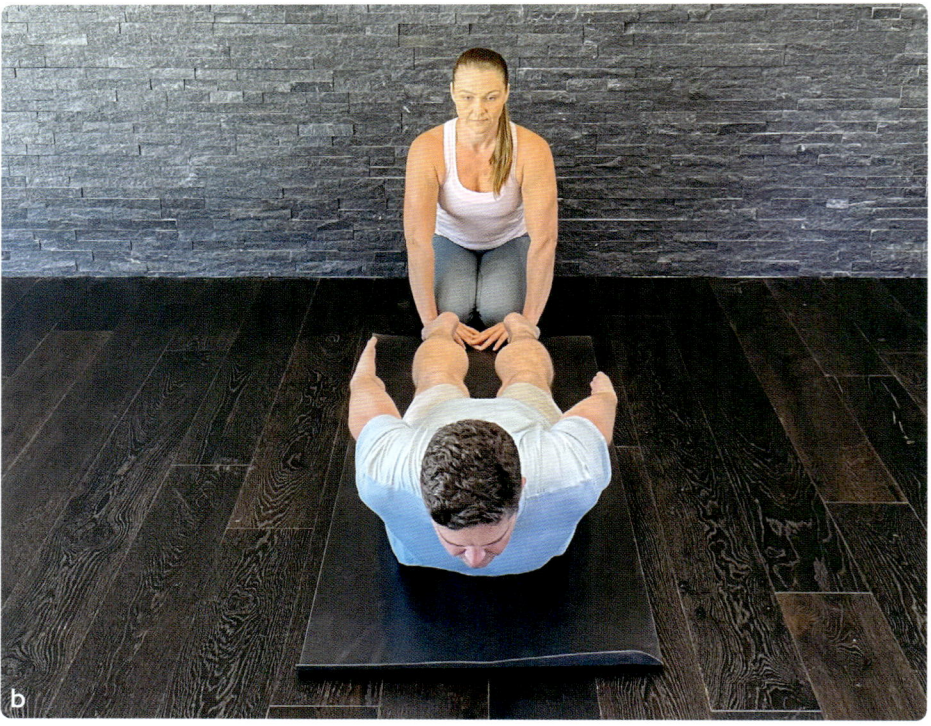

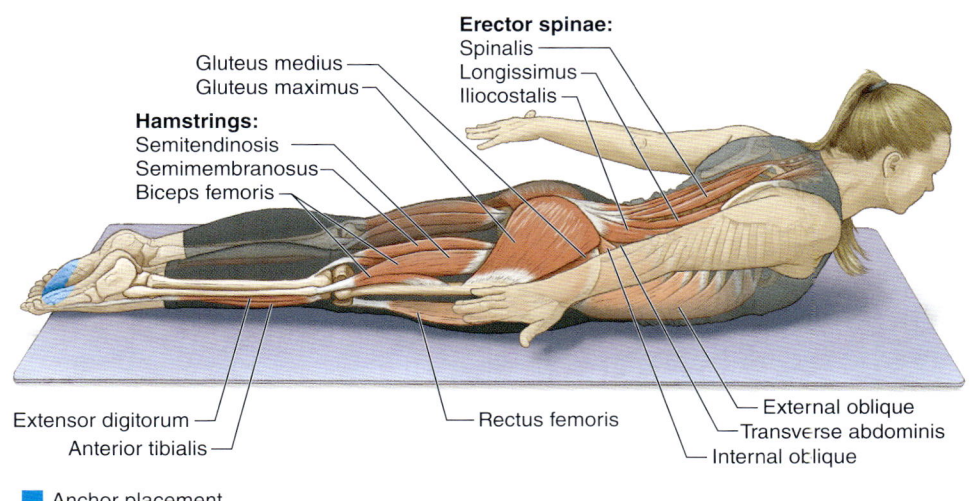

Erector spinae:
Spinalis
Longissimus
Iliocostalis

Gluteus medius
Gluteus maximus

Hamstrings:
Semitendinosis
Semimembranosus
Biceps femoris

Extensor digitorum
Anterior tibialis

Rectus femoris

External oblique
Transverse abdominis
Internal oblique

■ Anchor placement

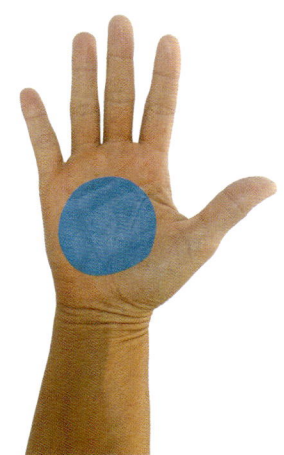

Anchor tool

STUDENT ALIGNMENT

Salabhasana: Locust Pose

The tops of the feet are on the ground, with all 10 toes rooting into the mat.

The arches of the feet are touching, or the feet are farther apart.

The kneecaps are lifted, and the thighs are firm.

The spine is in extension, with the chin in neutral.

The arms are in any variation suitable for the student.

Purpose

There are many variations of locust pose. In this variation, the student aims to root the tops of their feet into the mat, including all 10 toes. By grounding the feet, the student can better recruit their posterior chain and find greater spinal extension and a deeper backbend. An assist to the feet also supports a greater sense of grounding and support.

Stance

Kneeling

Alternative: Low Squat

Place your grounded knee just behind your student's feet. Using your legs, rock your weight forward so that your shoulders stack over your wrists and the student's feet. Your arms should remain straight throughout the assist.

Anchor Tool: Whole Palm of Both Hands

Turn your palms down, and angle your hands inward so that your fingers point toward each other.

Anchor Placement: Metatarsal Heads, Balls of Both Feet

Place one hand on each foot at the balls of the student's feet. If the feet are close together, you can stack the fingers of one hand on top of the other.

Stretch Placement: Provided by the Student

When the instructor provides more anchoring in this pose, the student can create greater spinal extension. As a result, they will feel more stretch along the anterior (front side) of their body, especially along the abdomen and torso.

Follow the Lines

The direction of pressure is directly down to the floor, mimicking the actions of this pose.

Myofascial Region

During contraction, this assist involves the myofascia of the spinal erectors, gluteals, hamstrings, anterior tibialis, and extensor digitorum muscles. During stretch, this assist involves the myofascia of the hip flexors (psoas, iliacus, rectus femoris) and abdominal muscles.

General Precautions

The floor is a hard surface, so a little goes a long way when pressing directly down toward the floor. Allow your pressure to be just enough to resist the student's feet from lifting off the floor.

Common Misalignments

If the student is practicing a variation of locust pose with their feet lifted, this is not the assist to offer. Teach the variation where the feet and all 10 toes remain rooted to the floor.

Troubleshooting

Be mindful that the anchoring pressure occurs at the balls of the feet and not at the ankles. Depending on the flexibility of the student's ankle, there may be a large curve between their ankle and the floor. You do not want to press down on this curve, compressing the foot into plantar flexion (or flattening the top of the foot to the floor), because it may hurt their ankle. Stay on the ball of the foot where the top of the foot (dorsal side) is fully contacting the floor.

This is an assist that I like to start just before a student comes into the pose. Set up for the assist by lightly placing your hands on the student's feet. Cue the entire room to root all 10 toes into the mat and lift their kneecaps. Apply slow, steady anchoring pressure directly downward. Then, instruct students to lift their chests into locust pose. Stay with the assist throughout the pose; don't assist multiple students unless you are teaching the pose multiple times. Once the student has brought their chest back to the mat and released the pose, slowly release the assist.

This assist can also be offered in low or high cobra poses.

If you are weaving work involving the feet into your sequence, it's a good idea to have hand sanitizer at your mat. After working with feet, if you're going to touch other parts of your students' bodies, give your hands a spritz first.

PUTTING IT ALL TOGETHER

- Find a kneeling stance just behind your student's feet.
- Before placing your hands on your student's feet, use your legs to bring your shoulders over the balls of their feet. If needed, modify your distance from the student to enable this movement.
- Turn both palms down and angle the hands inward. Place the palm of each hand on the ball of each foot.
- Using your legs, rock your weight forward to apply pressure directly down toward the floor. Be mindful that your shoulders stack directly over the wrists and your arms remain straight.
- When applying pressure, avoid being too forceful; only offer enough pressure to resist the lifting of the student's feet as they hold their backbend.
- Hold the assist for the duration the student holds the pose.
- Once the student brings their chest to the mat and returns to a resting position, slowly release both hands from the feet and step out of their space.

9
THIGH AND HIP

Child's Pose: Hip Press
Child's Pose: Sacral Press
Child's Pose: Thigh Rotation
Wide-Leg Forward Fold: Thigh Rotation

Child's Pose: Hip Press

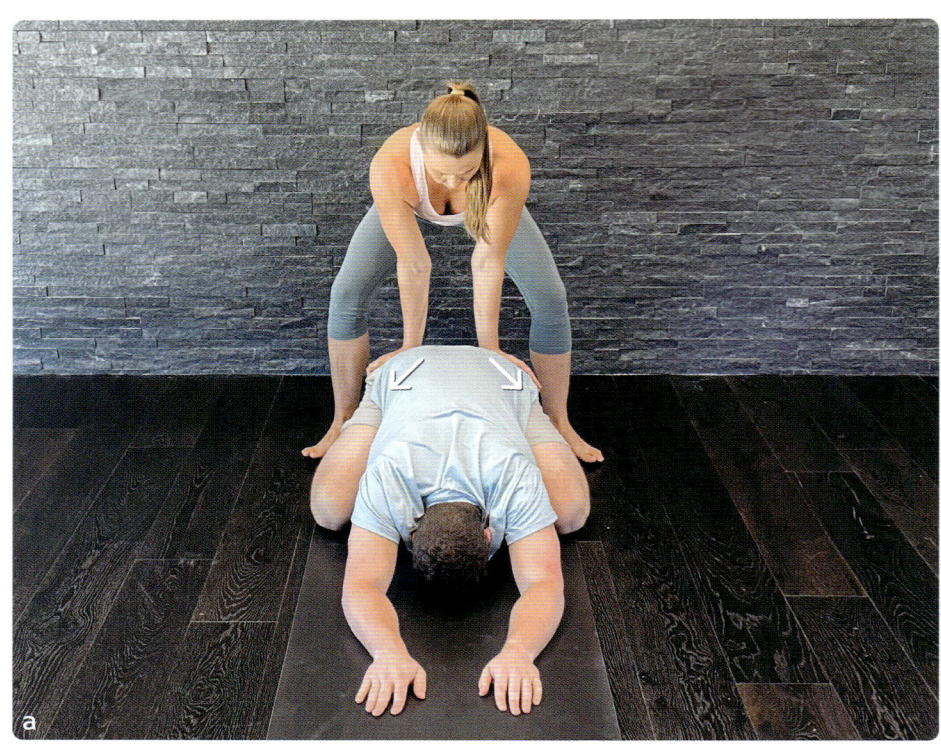

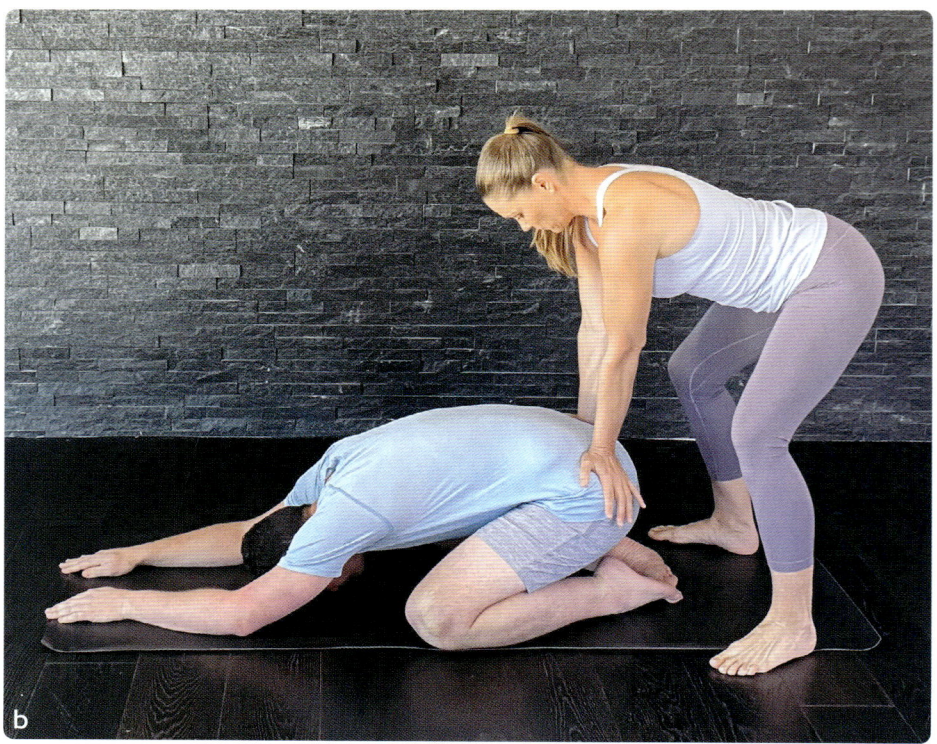

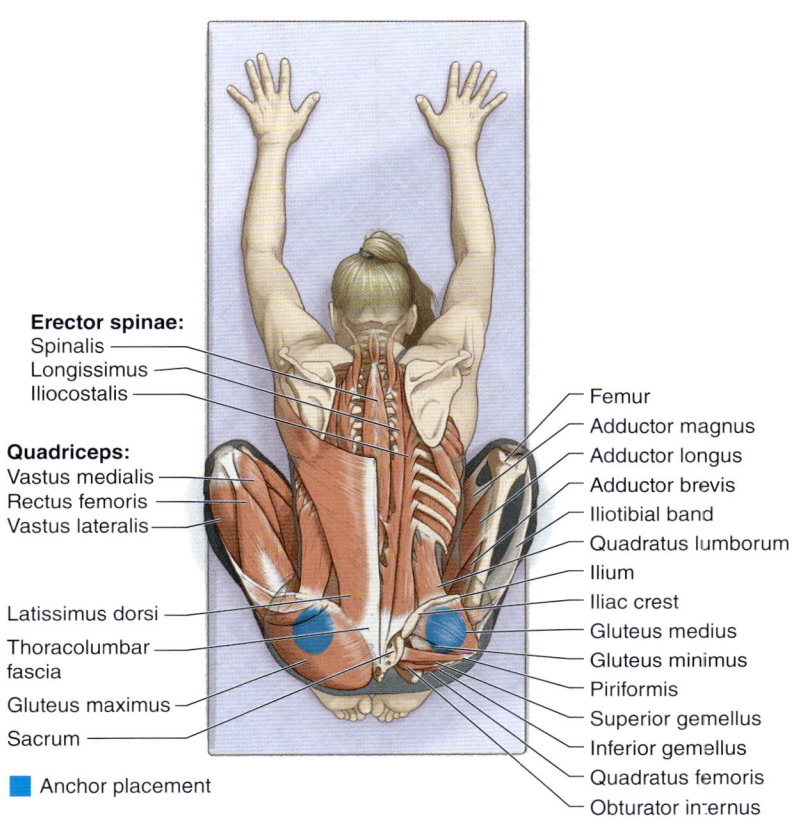

Erector spinae:
Spinalis
Longissimus
Iliocostalis

Quadriceps:
Vastus medialis
Rectus femoris
Vastus lateralis

Latissimus dorsi

Thoracolumbar fascia

Gluteus maximus

Sacrum

Femur
Adductor magnus
Adductor longus
Adductor brevis
Iliotibial band
Quadratus lumborum
Ilium
Iliac crest
Gluteus medius
Gluteus minimus
Piriformis
Superior gemellus
Inferior gemellus
Quadratus femoris
Obturator internus

■ Anchor placement

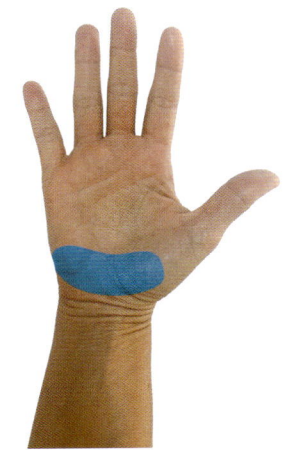

Anchor tool

Purpose

This assist offers greater grounding while also providing added stretch across the back of the hips. The hips are in flexion in wide-leg child's pose, which naturally stretches the gluteus maximus muscles. This assist emphasizes the stretch to these muscles, nearby tissues of the lower back, and adductor muscles of the inner thighs.

Stance

High Squat

Place your heels roughly outside of your student's toes. Based on your height, make sure that when you bend your knees and send your hips back, your shoulders stack directly over the student's hips and over your wrists. Your arms remain straight throughout the assist.

Anchor Tool: The Heel of Both Hands and Palm

Turn your palms down, then angle your hands so your fingers point toward 4 o'clock and 8 o'clock. Most of the pressure will come from the heel of your hand, though the entire palm will make contact with the glute. Keep your fingers softly lifted off the student's buttocks and directed outward to the right and left.

Anchor Placement: Gluteus Maximus Muscles

Once you are comfortable identifying the sacrum, move on to this assist that applies pressure directly to the gluteus maximus muscles just lateral to (to the right and left of) the sacrum. The gluteus maximus muscles are located just inferior to (below) the line of the waistband and just lateral to the T-shaped stitching on your student's pants (the area where the waistband meets the perpendicular center seam of their pants) found over the sacrum.

Place the heels of each hand on the gluteus maximus muscles just to the right and left of the sacrum. Be sure that when you apply pressure, you are not on the iliac crest or hip bones; your hands should be placed entirely on soft gluteal tissue just below the iliac crest.

Stretch Placement: Provided by the Student

The student will feel added stretch along the tops of the thighs and the inner thighs, glutes muscles, and low back. The more a student walks their hands towards the top of the mat, the greater a stretch can be felt.

Follow the Lines

The lines you're following are those of the gluteus maximus muscles, which originate at the ilium and sacrum and run lateroinferiorly (outward and downward) toward the femur (thigh bone). Direct the pressure down and out, toward the long edges of the student's mat. The pressure is not directly down toward the floor but at an angle outward and slightly downward. You can apply pressure with both hands simultaneously or alternate applying pressure with one hand and then the other. I often do a combination of the two if I am offering a longer assist.

Should you opt to alternate pressure, begin by pressing down and out with both hands to establish the anchor. To alternate pressure, maintain the anchor in one hand as you release the pressure in your opposite hand without removing your hand from the student. Remember to use your legs by shifting your weight into the foot that's maintaining the anchor pressure. When you shift sides, shift your body weight into the opposite foot while simultaneously applying the anchor pressure to the opposite side and releasing pressure from the previous hand.

Myofascial Region

The gluteus maximus receives the greatest stretch in this assist, although the deeper external rotators of the hip will feel the compression of this assist too. Depending on how tight a student's lower back and torso are, they may feel an additional stretch in the thoracolumbar region. Some students will experience greater stretch to the quadriceps and adductor muscles of the thighs, as well as the latissimus dorsi muscle, which may be felt on the posterior side of the axilla or armpit.

General Precautions

The hips can generally receive a lot of pressure if there are no injuries, pain, or previous surgeries to the region. Do not strain to apply a tremendous amount of pressure, but feel confident that you can apply a firm touch here. As you learn this assist, ask your students how the pressure feels.

Be careful to stay just inferior to (below) the iliac crest of the ilium (pelvic bones). Too low can feel too intimate, and it is! You will know you have the correct position if you feel only soft tissue just below the iliac crest.

This assist may not be appropriate to use in trauma-informed yoga settings.

Common Misalignments

The knees and ankles are the joints that can be commonly stressed by this assist. If a student cannot bring their hips near their heels, do not offer this assist to the student. If a student has their toes tucked to help reduce the plantar flexion through their ankles, do not offer this assist.

If the student is in traditional child's pose with the knees together and under the torso, this assist should not be provided as the handholds won't be adequate to offer the assist.

Troubleshooting

Because this assist can include a type of palpation—pressing one heel of the hand down into the gluteus maximus and then the other—feel free to use the back-and-forth motion to palpate with the heel of your hand to find the right spot. Use lighter pressure, as though providing the assist, to find the appropriate handholds where you will provide greater pressure. The intention of slowly palpating for the ideal location is to find the placement that feels like only soft tissue just below the iliac crest. This spot is similar for all students, so practice with people you are comfortable receiving feedback from on the correct hand placement.

PUTTING IT ALL TOGETHER

- Step into the student's space and find a high-squat stance, roughly aligning your heels with their toes.
- With your eyes, find the sacrum or the T-shaped stitching of their yoga bottoms, which indicates the general region of the sacrum.
- Turn your palms down and angle your fingers outward so that they point toward your feet.
- Place the heels of each hand on the student's glutes a few inches to the right and left of the sacrum or T-shaped stitching. Be mindful not to be "handsy" by lightly lifting your fingers away from their glutes.
- With shoulders over the wrists and arms straight, begin to bend your knees to transmit the strength of your legs into both hands.
- Apply pressure to both hips downward and out at an angle. The angle is toward your feet or the long edges of the mat.
- Apply pressure back and forth to either hip, or press both hips simultaneously and hold for a few moments.
- To complete the assist, begin to slowly straighten your knees to reduce pressure from the hands.
- Pause to ensure the student's hips have returned to their natural resting position before releasing both hands simultaneously.

Child's Pose: Sacral Press

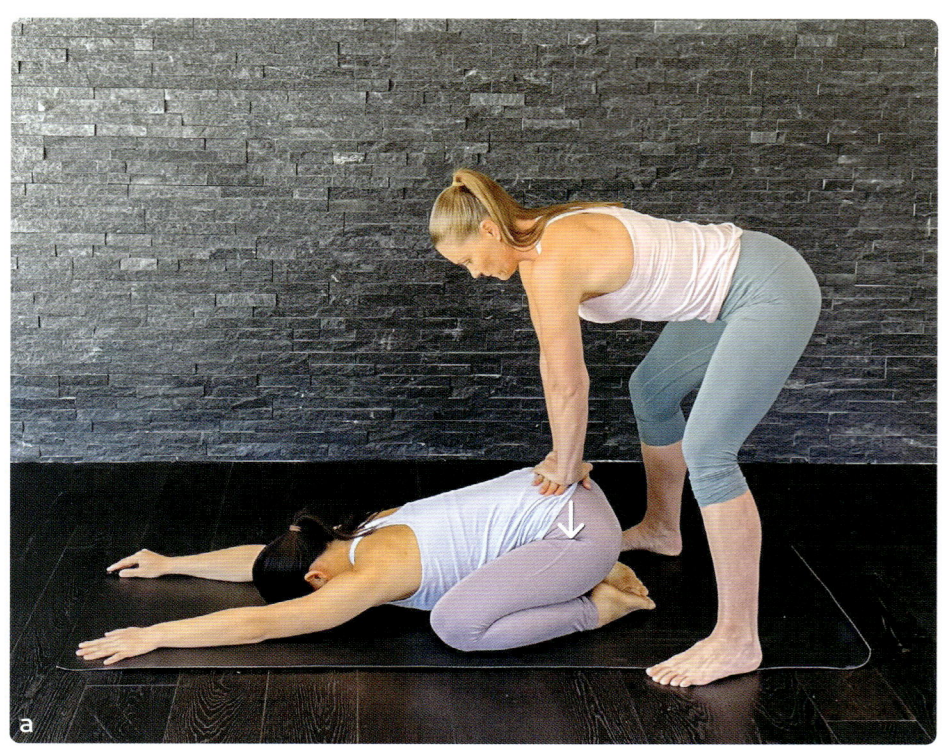

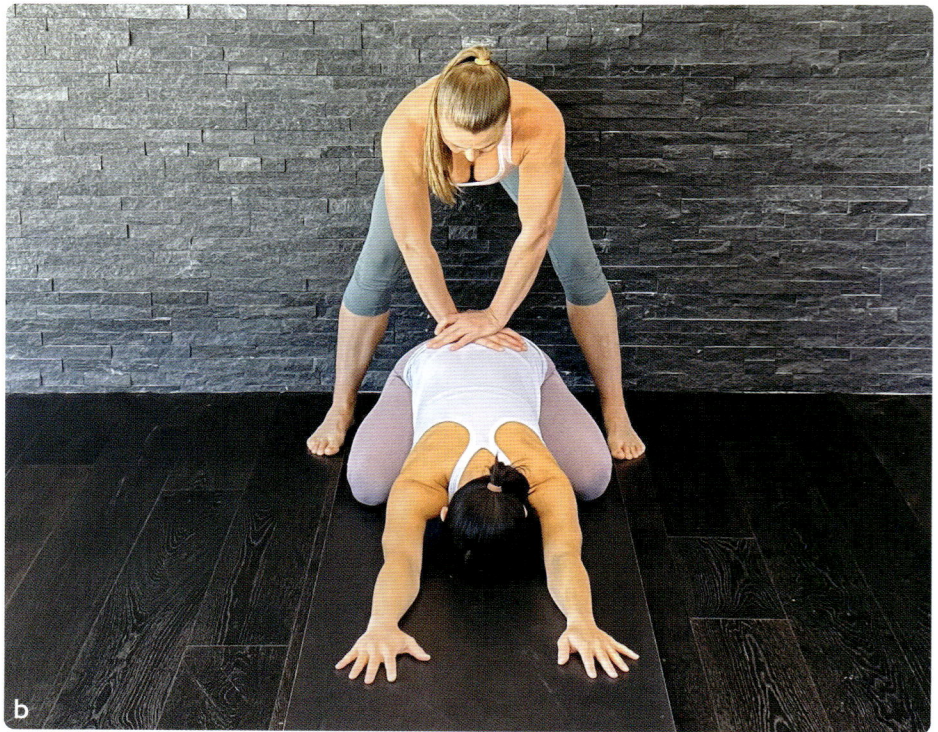

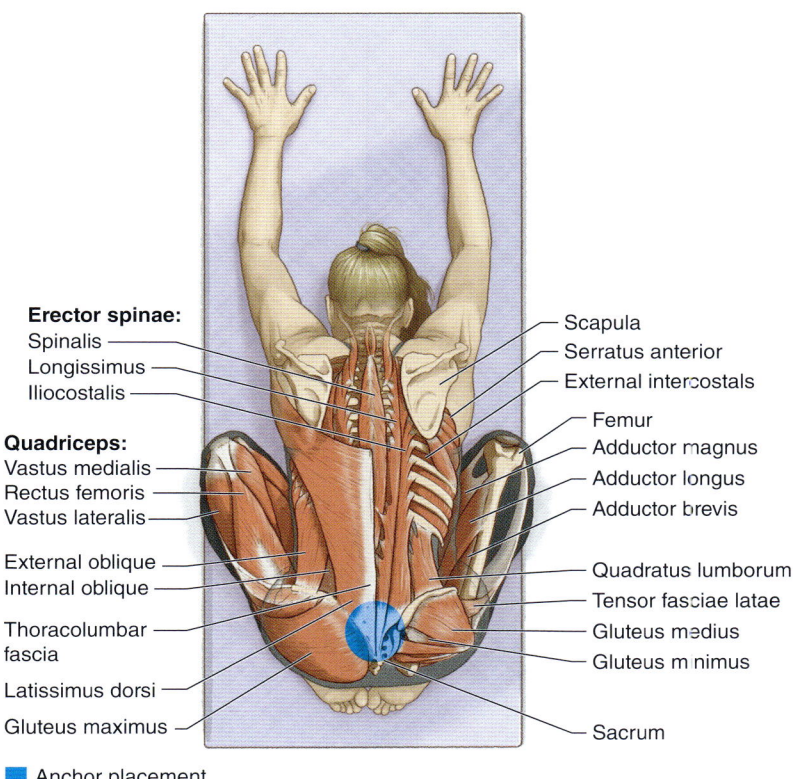

Erector spinae:
Spinalis
Longissimus
Iliocostalis

Quadriceps:
Vastus medialis
Rectus femoris
Vastus lateralis

External oblique
Internal oblique

Thoracolumbar fascia

Latissimus dorsi

Gluteus maximus

Scapula
Serratus anterior
External intercostals

Femur
Adductor magnus
Adductor longus
Adductor brevis

Quadratus lumborum
Tensor fasciae latae
Gluteus medius
Gluteus minimus

Sacrum

Anchor placement

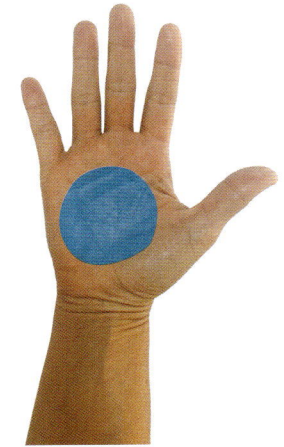

Anchor tool

STUDENT ALIGNMENT

Balasana: Wide-Leg Child's Pose

The big toes touch or are near one another.

The knees are placed wider than the torso.

The hips sink back toward the heels (they don't have to touch).

The torso rests passively between the thighs.

The forehead rests against the mat.

The arms lengthen toward the top of the mat.

The student appears still and comfortable.

Purpose

This is a passive pose because the student isn't working to bring their hips toward the heels once they've found the pose. When the teacher offers the sacral press, the student's hips sink farther toward the heels, and they feel a greater stretch along the spine and the tops of the thighs.

Stance

High Squat

Roughly align your heels with your student's toes. Based on your height, be sure that when you bend your knees and send your hips back, your shoulders stack over the wrists and the student's sacrum. Your arms remain straight throughout the assist. Bending the knees provides the strength in the assist.

Anchor Tool: Center of Palm

You can use one hand to offer this assist or stack your hands and use both. Turn your palms down, then angle your hands inward so that your fingers point toward the midline of the student's body. If using both hands, the palms will stack.

Anchor Placement

Look for the sacrum to apply the sacral press. Often, the sacrum falls beneath the T-shaped stitching of the student's pants. This is where the waistband meets the perpendicular center seam of their pants. You know you have found the sacrum when you feel a bone at the center of the hips that is slightly convex (rounded toward you). Place your palm directly over the sacrum, with your fingers pointing inward or toward the midline of the body.

Stretch Placement: Provided by the Student

The student's outstretched arms create the stretch point in this assist. The more a student reaches their fingers forward and plants their palms down, the more they will feel the stretch along their spine and torso.

Follow the Lines

The hips are sinking toward the heels in child's pose. This assist mimics the sinking of the hips by applying the pressure in the assist directly downward toward the floor.

Myofascial Region

This assist includes all myofascia that runs adjacent to the spine, especially the spinal erectors, the quadratus lumborum, and the thoracolumbar fascia of the lower back. The more the student lengthens through the arms, the more they will feel the stretch along the lateral body or sides of the torso—namely, the abdominal obliques, intercostal muscles, serratus anterior, and latissimus dorsi. The quadriceps will also feel a stretch as the sacral press creates greater flexion through the hips and knees.

General Precautions

The hips can generally receive a lot of pressure. Do not strain to apply a tremendous amount of pressure, but feel confident that you can apply a firm touch here. As you learn this assist, ask your students how the pressure feels. Do not offer this assist to any student with a known hip issue.

Common Misalignments

The knees and ankles are the joints that can be commonly stressed by this assist. If a student cannot bring their hips to their heels, do not offer this assist to the student. If a student has their toes tucked to help reduce the plantar flexion of their ankles, do not offer this assist.

If the student is in traditional child's pose with the knees together and under the torso, this assist is not ideal to provide. With the knees together, the tailbone and sacrum tuck under as the spine is put into greater flexion. With the tailbone tucked under, it's more difficult to access and increases the chance of your hand slipping, making the handhold unstable.

Troubleshooting

The sacral press is applied directly to bone. Locate the pronounced, rounded bone at the base of the spine. Avoid pressing straight down on the lower back or placing your hands so low that you feel the natal cleft or tailbone. The sacrum is a solid, stable bone, and your handhold should remain on this structure.

PUTTING IT ALL TOGETHER

- Step into the student's space and find a high-squat stance, roughly aligning your heels with your student's toes.
- With your eyes, find the sacrum or the T-shaped stitching of their yoga bottoms; the spot where the stitching intersects is usually where you will find the sacrum.
- Making sure that your spine stays straight, stack your shoulders over your wrists as you place your palm(s) on the student's sacrum.
- The sacrum feels slightly convex or rounded; place the center of your palm on this bone. Adjust your hand placement as needed to find the sacrum.
- Be sure your shoulders are over the student's sacrum, your arms are straight, and you feel a rounded bone beneath your palm(s).
- Moving slowly, bend your knees to apply pressure straight down toward the floor until you feel the resistance or density in the tissues—this is their limit.
- Hold the downward pressure of the assist for a few moments.
- To complete the assist, begin to slowly straighten your knees and reduce pressure on the sacrum until your student's hips return to their natural resting position.
- Pause to ensure the student's tissues have returned to their natural resting position before releasing your hand(s) and stepping out of the student's space.

Child's Pose: Thigh Rotation

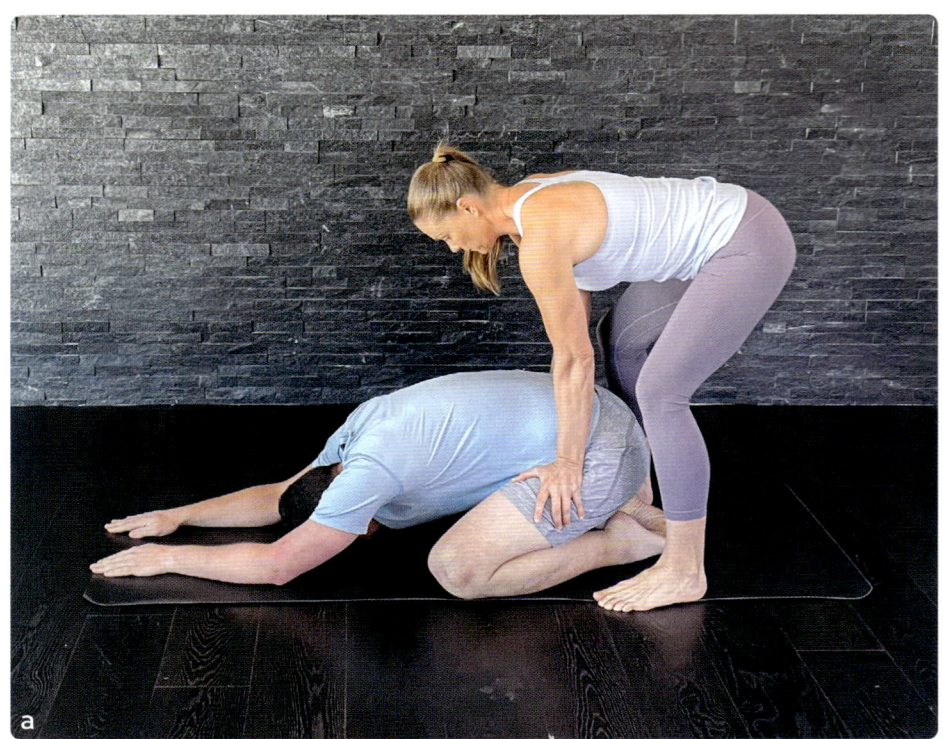

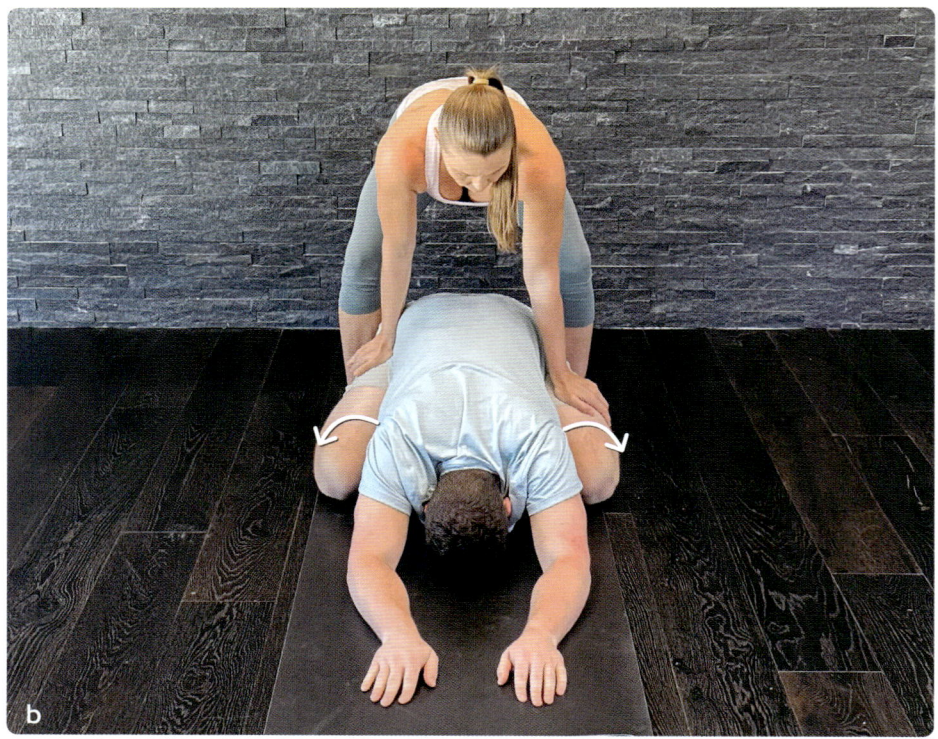

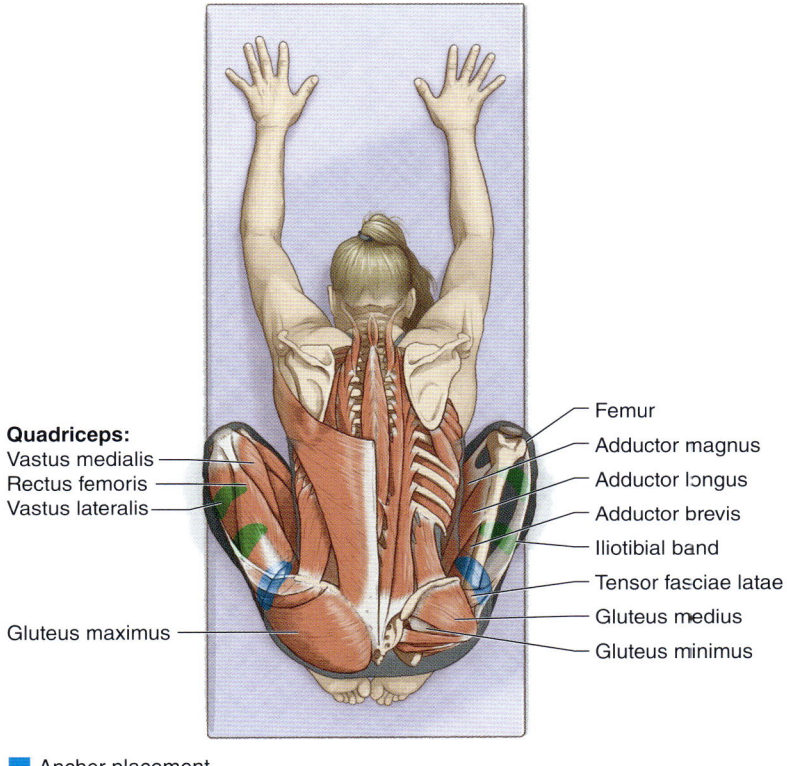

Quadriceps:
Vastus medialis
Rectus femoris
Vastus lateralis

Gluteus maximus

Femur
Adductor magnus
Adductor longus
Adductor brevis
Iliotibial band
Tensor fasciae latae
Gluteus medius
Gluteus minimus

■ Anchor placement
■ Dynamic stretch placement

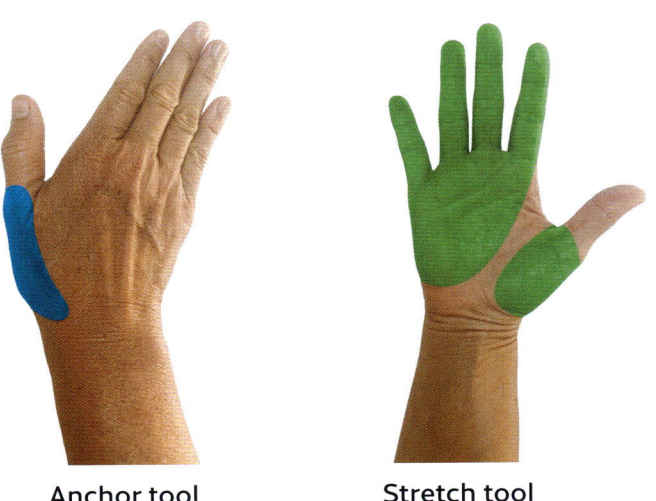

Anchor tool

Stretch tool

Purpose

Wide-leg child's pose is technically a hip-opening pose. The wider the student places their knees, the greater the stretch to the adductors of the inner thighs. By rotating the myofascia externally in this assist, you're mimicking the hip opening of the pose and heightening the sense of stretch felt in the adductor muscles of the inner thighs.

Stance

High Squat

Roughly align your heels with your student's toes. Based on your height, be sure that when you bend your knees and send your hips back, your shoulders stack over your wrists and the student's upper thighs. Your arms should be straight throughout the assist. Shift your weight between your feet as you apply pressure back and forth to each thigh.

Anchor Tool: Thenar Eminence (Base of Thumb) and Entire Palmar Surface of Hand

The tool is important in this assist. The base of the thumb finds and wedges into the uppermost hip crease first. Keep your fingers lifted until you place the thenar eminence in the hip crease. Once you've snuggly placed your thumb base in the hip crease, allow your fingers to lightly rest on the thigh and your entire palm to sink into their tissue.

Anchor Placement: Proximal Thigh, Upper Quadriceps

Start the assist by establishing the initial anchor at the outer hip creases. Place the base of your thumb in the student's hip crease. This is the angle and fold of clothing where the thigh meets the hip.

To place your thumb at the outer hip crease, start from the angle of the thigh. That is, don't place your hand from above. Instead, bring the base of your thumb on the thigh about two to three inches (5-7 cm) below the hip crease. Contact the thighs with the base of your thumbs. Slide the base of your thumbs up the short distance of the thighs, and then snugly sink your thumb bases into the outer hip creases. This is like scooping into the hip creases.

Depending on the student, their torso may be in contact with the inner thighs, and you may need to almost wedge the base of your thumbs into the outer hip creases. This is okay to do. It feels best to receive this assist if the teacher begins with this initial anchor by pressing both hip creases simultaneously.

Try this to make your thenar eminence more pronounced: Turn your palm down, then angle your fingers outward. This will bring the base of the thumb forward while also pointing your thumb tip away (as shown in the anchor tool image). At the base of your thumb, there is a rounded bone (metacarpal) where your thumb meets your wrist. This is the portion of your thumb you want to place snuggly in the student's hip crease. Use the previously described wrist alignment before placing your hands on your student.

Stretch Tool: Thenar Eminence (Base of Thumb) and Entire Palmar Surface of Hand

The stretch tool is identical to the anchor tool. The hands will alternate back and forth with one hand statically anchoring while the other moves down the opposite thigh and dynamically externally rotates the thigh tissue. The hand externally rotating the thigh is the stretch; the hand providing a static counterbalance or stabilization is the anchor.

Without grabbing or curling your fingertips into the student's tissues, sink the entire palmar surface and fingers into the thigh tissue in order to roll the tissue outward. Think about the tool being a broad surface to move more of the thigh tissue.

Stretch Placement: Quadriceps

After establishing the initial anchor, keep one hand at the outer hip crease applying downward pressure; this hand remains the anchor. With the opposite hand, move down the high towards the knee an inch or two. Sink the whole hand into the thigh tissue (without grabbing or using fingertips) and dynamically rotate the tissue outward. Depending on the tissue, there may be very little external rotation to the tissue. That's okay, listen for the bounds of their tissue and stop when you feel it resist or pull back. When you feel this bound, maintain the pressure and hold your hand here to now make this hand the anchor. With the opposite hand that was previously the anchor, slide down the thigh a few inches and repeat the action of dynamically rotating the tissue out and holding. The dynamic movement is the stretch, the static pressure is the anchor. Alternate back and forth, shifting your weight into the leg that matches the hand that's dynamically moving to stretch and then anchor.

Follow the Lines

The directional pressure in this assist is twofold, first downward toward the floor and then externally rotating along the thigh. The downward pressure at the hip creases mimics the hips sinking toward the heels, and the external rotation of the thighs follows the hip opening of the thighs.

Once both bases of the thumbs have hooked into each hip crease, apply pressure downward toward the floor, allowing your whole hand to sink into the tissues. Do not aim to squeeze the student's thighs with your hands. Instead, simply allow your whole hand to sink into their tissues to get a full handhold.

After the initial press downward at the hip crease, maintain the downward pressure with one hand, and with the other hand, roll the tissue of the quadriceps externally, away from the torso. Alternate pressure back and forth; one hand stabilizes while the other hand rolls the thigh tissue away. Work your way down each thigh toward the knees, pressing into the tissue and rolling out.

After you have rolled the tissue outward with each hand and are a few inches above the knee, slide the base of each thumb back to the hip crease and apply one final downward press to both hip creases.

To recap, you will press at the hip crease with both hands, externally rotate each thigh two to three times down the length of the thigh, and then finish with a final press with both hands at the hip creases.

Myofascial Region

The external rotation of the thighs directly stretches the adductors of the inner thighs. The student will feel compression along the quadriceps and iliotibial band of the thighs, as well as at the tensor fascia latae, gluteus medius, and gluteus minimus at the hip crease. Similar to other child's pose assists, the more the student chooses to lengthen towards the top of their mat, the more of a stretch they'll feel along the torso.

General Precautions

Avoid trying to forcibly roll the tissue of the thigh outward near the knee. This will create rotational stress near the knee joint and would be uncomfortable for the student. Pressure directly towards the kneecap is fine, however forcibly rotating the tissue away from the knee must be avoided; lighten your pressure here.

Avoid overthinking the fact that you're using your whole hand to externally rotate the myofascia of the thigh. If you aren't clawing or sinking your fingertips into your student, you're probably doing it correctly. The idea is to have a broad, flat surface to rotate as much thigh tissue as possible.

This assist may not be appropriate to use in trauma-informed yoga settings.

Common Misalignments

The knees and ankles are the common joints that can be stressed by this assist. If a student cannot bring their hips to their heels, do not offer this assist to the student. If a student has their toes tucked to help reduce the plantar flexion of their ankles, do not offer this assist.

If a student has their knees apart, but not wide enough for you to readily access the tops of the thighs, the student should not be provided this assist. Of course, this assist cannot be provided to students who are holding a traditional child's pose with the knees together and held under the torso, as handholds are not accessible.

Troubleshooting

The higher you can place the base of your thumb in the hip crease, the better. This is a visible location you can easily view from above, but sometimes you must wedge your thumb pad into the crease for access. Teachers in training will sometimes avoid doing this because they misconstrue it as invasive. Because the hip crease sits entirely on the outer (lateral) hip, it isn't experienced as invasive when you hook your thumb pad into it. It also feels the best when the hip crease is accessed. Practice finding the hip crease with friends and receive feedback on your placement. You'll know you have it when it feels like your thumb pad has fully hooked into the hip crease.

PUTTING IT ALL TOGETHER

- Step into the student's space, roughly align your heels with the student's toes, and find a high-squat stance.
- Turn your palms down and angle your fingers outward, bringing the base of your thumb forward.
- Keep your back and arms straight as you bend your knees to place the base of your thumbs on the student's upper thighs a couple of inches below the hip creases.
- Slide the base of your thumbs as high up into the outer hip creases as you can access. Your thumbs and fingers point outward and softly lift.
- Allow your fingers to rest on the student's thighs, but do not grip with the fingertips. Gently sink your whole hand into each thigh. Do not squeeze.
- With your shoulders over the wrists and your arms straight, begin to bend your knees to transmit the strength of your legs into the base of both thumbs, pressing both hip creases directly downward.
- Sliding one hand down the thigh, without squeezing the student's tissues, roll their flesh externally (outward), away from the midline of the body. The opposite hand maintains the downward anchor pressure.
- Alternate hands. After rolling one thigh, pause and hold the down-and-out pressure. Slide the other hand down a few inches, roll the tissue down and out, and pause while maintaining the anchor pressure. Slide the other hand down and repeat the previous motions.
- Work your way from the hip crease to the knee, but stop rolling the tissue outward a few inches above the knee.
- To finish the assist, slide both thumb bases back up to the hip creases and provide one final press toward the floor. Slowly lift both hands and return the student's hips to their natural resting position before removing both hands simultaneously.

Wide-Leg Forward Fold: Thigh Rotation

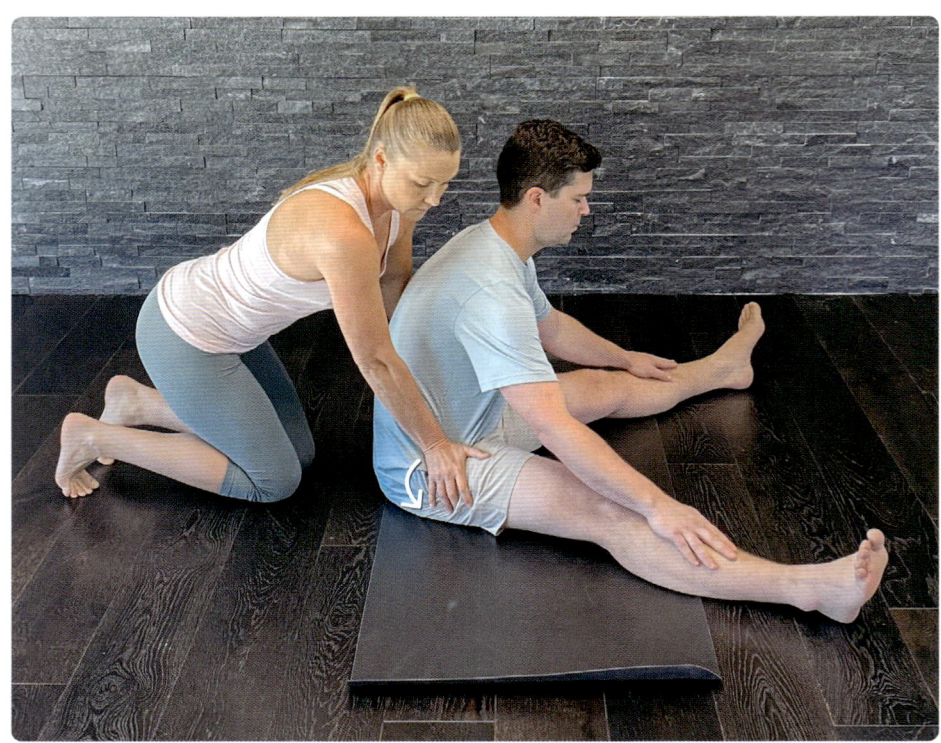

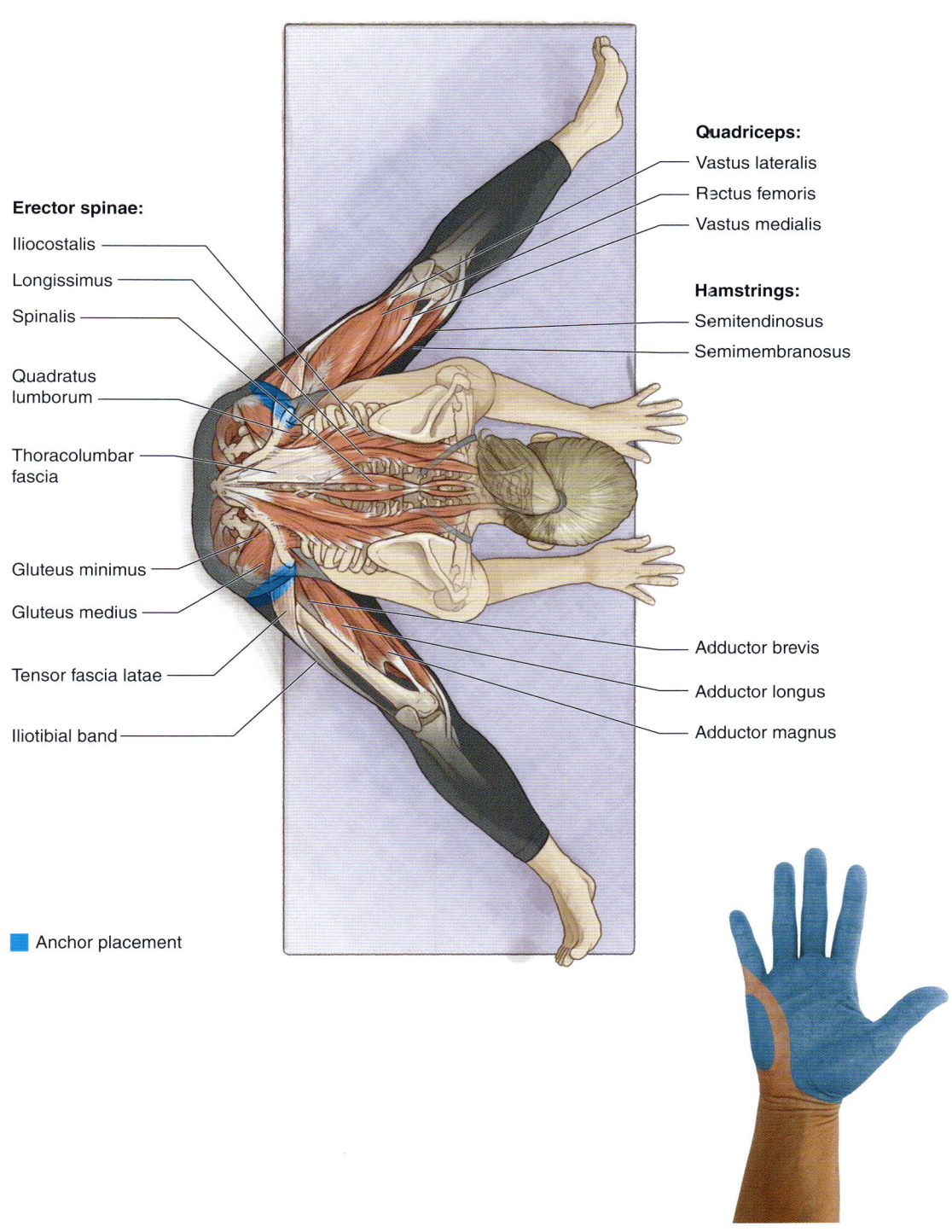

Quadriceps:

Vastus lateralis

Rectus femoris

Vastus medialis

Hamstrings:

Semitendinosus

Semimembranosus

Erector spinae:

Iliocostalis

Longissimus

Spinalis

Quadratus lumborum

Thoracolumbar fascia

Gluteus minimus

Gluteus medius

Tensor fascia latae

Iliotibial band

Adductor brevis

Adductor longus

Adductor magnus

■ Anchor placement

Anchor tool

STUDENT ALIGNMENT

Upavistha Konasana: Seated Wide-Leg Forward-Fold Pose

The hips are resting evenly on the mat or a low prop (such as a blanket).

The feet are wide (as suitable for each individual student).

The legs and feet are relaxed in yin or restorative classes; in active vinyasa-style classes, the legs and feet are engaged, with the feet dorsiflexed.

The spine is straight from the tailbone to the crown of the head.

The torso is folded forward between the thighs.

The hands or forearms rest on the floor, legs, or a prop.

Purpose

The action of this pose is to anchor the hips and forward fold. The more a student can emphasize both actions, the more stretch they will experience in the spinal erectors, hamstrings, and adductor muscles. The assist adds to the action of the anchor, allowing the student to fold farther forward, if they so choose, to heighten the stretch in these muscle groups.

Stance

Kneeling

Wait until your student is fully in the pose before offering the assist. If they aren't folded forward, you won't be able to stack your shoulders over your wrists.

Place your knees behind your student, squaring your chest and shoulders to their back. Stand on your knees so that you can bring your chest over your wrists and the student's thighs. Your arms should remain straight throughout the assist.

Anchor Tool: Entire Palmar Surfaces of Hands

Turn your palms down, and angle your hands so that your thumbs point outward and your fingers point back toward you. Starting two to three inches (5-7 cm) away from the student's outer hip crease, slide the pinky edge of your hands up the thighs and snugly place the pinky edge of your palms into the outer hip creases. Starting two to three inches (5-7 cm) away allows you to scoop the pinky edges of your palms into the hip creases.

Anchor Placement: Proximal Quadriceps, Upper Thigh

The aim is to accentuate the grounding action of the hips. By placing your anchor as close to the outer hip creases as possible, you reinforce the feeling of the hips being anchored rather than the thighs. Contact the top of the thighs nearest the hips.

Stretch Placement: Provided by the Student

When the student is folded forward, walking their hands farther forward creates the added stretch to the adductors, hamstrings, and spinal erectors in this pose.

Follow the Lines

Apply pressure down toward the floor with a subtle outward rotation of the thighs, away from the student's midline. The directional pressure is directly downward, toward the floor, while also slightly encouraging externally rotating. This mimics the actions of the pose. The student passively externally rotates at the hips as they fold forward, but part of the effort is to anchor the hips as the torso lengthens forward.

Myofascial Region

This assist directly compresses the quadriceps of the thigh and the tensor fascia latae, gluteus medius, and gluteus minimus of the hip. Students will feel the added stretch in the pose in the adductors, hamstrings, spinal erectors, quadratus lumborum, and thoracolumbar fascia.

General Precautions

To keep a supported stance in this pose, the student must be folded forward. Be sure to start and end the assist before the student lifts their torso out of the pose.

This assist is generally safe for any student who doesn't have a hip condition. The assist only provides the anchor; the student determines how much added stretch they wish to experience by determining the depth of their forward fold.

This assist may not be appropriate to use in trauma-informed yoga settings.

Common Misalignments

If a student's torso is perpendicular to the floor, meaning they can't fold forward at all, this is not a student you should offer the assist to because you won't be able to stack your shoulders over your wrists to find a supported stance.

Troubleshooting

Be mindful that you offer this assist *at* the outer hip crease and not the upper portion of the thigh. You can think of the thigh bone (femur) as a lever. If you press at the most proximal end, at the hip crease, it's going to keep pressure away from the knee joint. The more you move away from the hip crease—down the thigh and closer to the knee—the more pressure will be placed on the knee, which is already in extension. Avoid applying pressure anywhere other than the uppermost thigh and outer hip crease.

If a student is sitting on a block or any other prop that elevates their hips without providing support along the back of the thigh, do not offer this assist. You do not want to offer this assist to students who have a gap between the backs of their thighs and the floor. Even if you apply pressure at the hip crease, when the thigh is elevated and not fully resting on something (a low blanket or the floor), the assist will apply undesirable pressure to the knee.

Be sure the student is aware of your presence before placing your hands on their thighs. If you're still cuing the class, they'll know you're there. Otherwise, rub your hands behind the student so that they are aware of your presence.

PUTTING IT ALL TOGETHER

- Ensure that your student is folded forward before offering this assist.
- Find a kneeling stance directly behind your student, squaring your hips and shoulders to their back.
- Standing on your knees, turn your palms down and position your hands so that the thumbs point out and your fingers point back toward you.
- Slide the pinky edge of your hand into your student's outer hip crease, being mindful that thumbs and fingers are pointing away from the student's midline and are on the outside of their thighs.
- Bring your chest forward and over the student to stack your shoulders over your wrists. Straighten your arms and apply pressure downward as you gently roll the myofascia of their thigh outward, or back toward you.
- With both hands holding the pressure in the assist, maintain pressure for a few moments or breaths.
- To release the assist, start to rock your weight back toward your feet and slowly lift both hands.
- Wait to cue the class to come out of this pose until you have exited the student's space.

10
SPINE

Child's Pose: Spinal Lengthening
Downward Dog: Front Press
Easy-Seat Side Stretch: Hip Anchor
Supine Twist: Spinal Lengthening
Deer Pose: Spinal Lengthening

Child's Pose: Spinal Lengthening

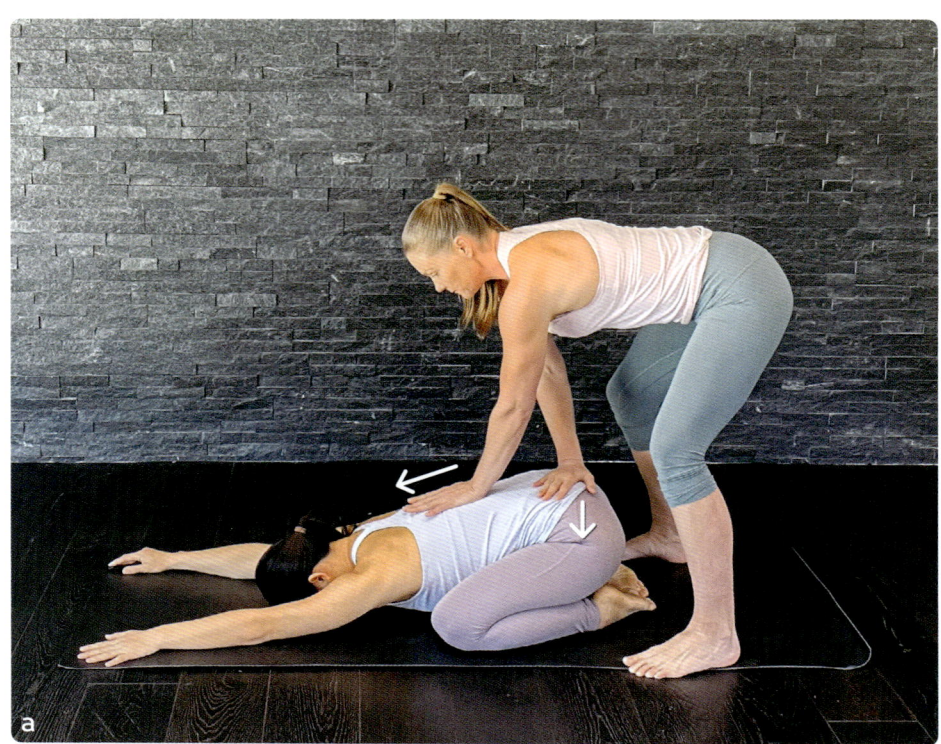

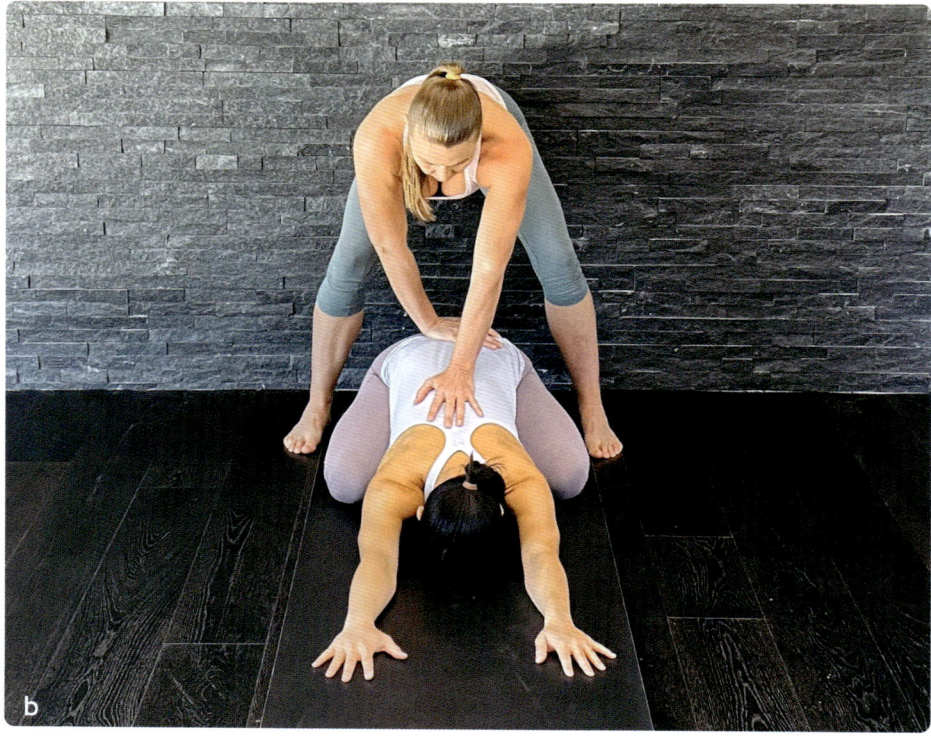

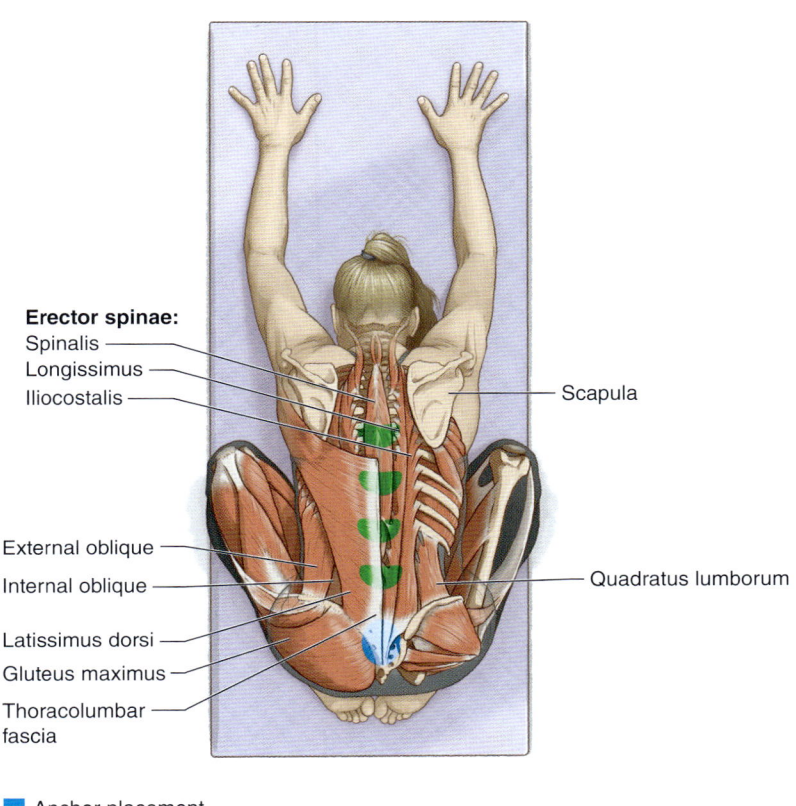

Erector spinae:
Spinalis
Longissimus
Iliocostalis

Scapula

External oblique

Internal oblique

Quadratus lumborum

Latissimus dorsi

Gluteus maximus

Thoracolumbar
fascia

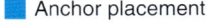
Anchor placement
Dynamic stretch placement

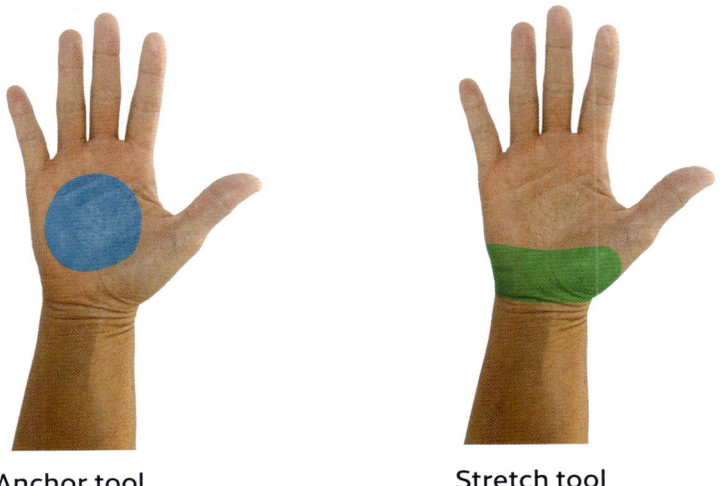

Anchor tool   Stretch tool

STUDENT ALIGNMENT

Balasana: Wide-Leg Child's Pose

The big toes touch or are near one another.
The knees are placed wider than the torso.
The hips sink back toward the heels (they don't have to touch).
The torso rests passively between the thighs.
The forehead rests against the mat.
The arms lengthen toward the top of the mat.
The student appears still and comfortable.

Purpose

Although wide-leg child's pose is a hip opener, it also provides stretch along the spine and torso via the hips sinking back and the arms lengthening forward. This assist supports both actions by offering more grounding to the sacrum and added stretch along the erectors of the spine.

Stance

High Squat

Roughly align your heels with your student's toes, but make sure to place your feet so that your shoulders stack over the hand you will use to place the anchor. Bend into the knees to recruit the strength of the legs to maintain downward pressure into the anchor throughout the assist. The opposite hand, the stretch hand, needs to provide only marginal pressure by comparison. With a straight spine, lean over the student so that your spine is roughly parallel to the floor. The opposite hand will reach long, along the student's spine, providing the stretch placement.

Anchor Tool: Palm of Dominant Hand

I encourage you to swap hands in this assist to find which hand feels the strongest for you as the anchor hand. Using the palm of your hand, turn your arm inward so your fingers point toward the midline of your body. Be mindful to keep your fingers softly lifted away from your student's body.

Anchor Placement: Sacrum

Place one palm on the rounded, convex bone of the sacrum. You will apply the anchor placement first. After you've applied the stretch placement along the length of the student's spine, you'll release this anchor placement last.

See Child's Pose: Sacral Press, page 138, for more information on this portion of the assist.

Stretch Tool: Heel of Opposite Hand

Use the heel of your hand to apply the pressure, and allow the rest of your hand to relax. You can even allow your fingers to rest lightly on the student's back rather than tensing your hand to keep the fingers lifted.

Stretch Placement: Spine and Spinal Erectors

You will place the stretch tool directly on the spine. Beginning at the lumbar region of the spine (low back), just ahead of your anchor hand, apply pressure at a few points along the spine between the lumbar region and shoulder blades. The spine becomes much more mobile at the shoulder blades, and pressing beyond this point may push the student's face into the floor. You also risk putting the outstretched arms into too much flexion at the shoulder joint. Stop palpating at about the line of the shoulder blades or at the point along the spine where you start to see the upper back and torso move beneath the pressure of your hand.

Follow the Lines

There are two actions in this pose that the anchor and the stretch mimic. The anchor mimics the action of the student's hips sinking toward the heels. The stretch mimics the elongation of the spine the student is creating as they extend their arms toward the top of the mat. The student isn't trying to sink their torso into the floor, so we don't want to press the student's spine into the floor with the stretch tool. The stretch tool follows the line along the spine, horizontal to the floor.

Apply the anchor first by placing your palm on the student's sacrum and pressing directly down toward the floor. Maintain consistent pressure throughout the assist. The anchor will be the last contact with the student.

Use the heel of the opposite hand to sink into your student's tissues. This is only the slightest pressure downward so that you feel as though you've hooked into the student's tissues for a secure handhold. Once you have sunk into their tissues, you apply the stretch by pressing the tissue superiorly toward the crown of the student's head.

Starting at the lumbar region, press up the spine with the stretch tool, creating a palpating motion. Sink into the student's tissues and press superiorly toward their head. Back out of the pressure to gently slide the heel of your hand up the spine a couple of inches. Then, gently sink back into the tissues, press superiorly again, slowly release pressure, slide the hand up, and repeat.

The lines of stretch are between your two hands, so let the action feel like you are pulling the tissue apart between the anchor and stretch placement.

Myofascial Region

The spinal erectors, quadratus lumborum, latissimus dorsi, and thoracolumbar fascia of the lower back are stretched in this assist.

General Precautions

Be mindful not to palpate too far up the spine. If a student has shoulder issues and you press firmly at the mid-thoracic or mid-spine level, it can create more flexion in the shoulder than the student is comfortable with. Be mindful to keep the pressure moving superiorly, up the spine, rather than pushing down toward the floor. Stop around the shoulder blades or when the student's spine begins to bend beneath your stretch hand.

Many students wear open-back shirts in yoga class. Do not offer this assist to a student who has an exposed back. If the upper back is partially exposed, I will offer this assist on the lower back and stop at the point where there is no more clothing. If their shirt has only hiked up a little bit, you can pull the shirt down and place it beneath the anchor tool, holding the clothing in place, to avoid touching skin.

Common Misalignments

This pose can commonly stress the joints of the knees and ankles. If a student cannot bring their hips towards their heels, do not offer this assist to the student. If a student has their toes tucked to help reduce the plantar flexion of their ankles, do not offer this assist.

If the student is in traditional child's pose with the knees together and under the torso, this assist is not ideal to provide. With the knees together, the tailbone and sacrum tuck under as the spine is put into greater flexion. With the tailbone tucked under, it's more difficult to access the sacrum and increases the chances of your hand slipping, making the anchor handhold unstable.

Troubleshooting

Most teachers make the mistake of being hyperfocused on their stretch hand and forget about their anchor hand. The anchor hand is what makes this assist feel good! If you keep the pressure firm and consistent in the anchor hand, you will need very little effort from the stretch hand. As you apply the stretch superiorly toward the crown of the head, you will feel the "rubber band" of their tissues provide feedback; the tissues between your two hands will become taut. When you feel that subtle stretch of tissue, you know you have it right.

When moving your stretch hand along the student's spine, don't remove your hand from their back entirely; just lift enough to slide your hand up the spine without dragging their tissues or clothing with you. Think of it as backing out of sinking into the tissues, just like a palpation.

It's easy for a student's shirt to lift in this assist. What I often do—and recommend to my trainees—is take the bottom of their shirt and pull it down over the sacrum as I start the assist. I then place my anchor hand on the shirt, as well as the sacrum. This holds the clothing in place as I elongate their spine, so I have no concern about touching skin.

PUTTING IT ALL TOGETHER

- Step into the student's space and find a high-squat stance with your heels roughly aligned with the student's toes.

- With your eyes, find the sacrum or the T-shaped stitching of their yoga bottoms. Where the stitching intersects is usually where you will find the sacrum.

- Making sure that your spine stays straight, stack your shoulders over your wrist as you place the palm of your anchor hand on the student's sacrum.

- With your arm straight, begin to bend your knees to press the sacrum directly down to the floor to establish the anchor.

- Maintain the downward pressure of the anchor on the sacrum for the duration of the assist.

- Begin at the lumbar spine. With the heel of your opposite hand, sink into your student's tissues by gently pushing into the spine (only enough to find traction), and then press up toward the head.

- As you maintain the downward anchor pressure, it will feel as though the stretch hand is lengthening the spinal tissues from the anchored sacrum. The stretch hand is lengthening the spine.

- Palpate up the spine with the heel of the stretch hand from the lower back to about the shoulder blades. Stop if you see the thoracic spine move or bounce beneath your hand.

- To complete the assist, simply hold your stretch hand a moment longer at about the region of the shoulder blades.

- Avoid the snapback by slowly releasing the stretch hand first and then the anchor hand, allowing the hips to return to their natural resting position before removing the anchor hand entirely.

Downward Dog: Front Press

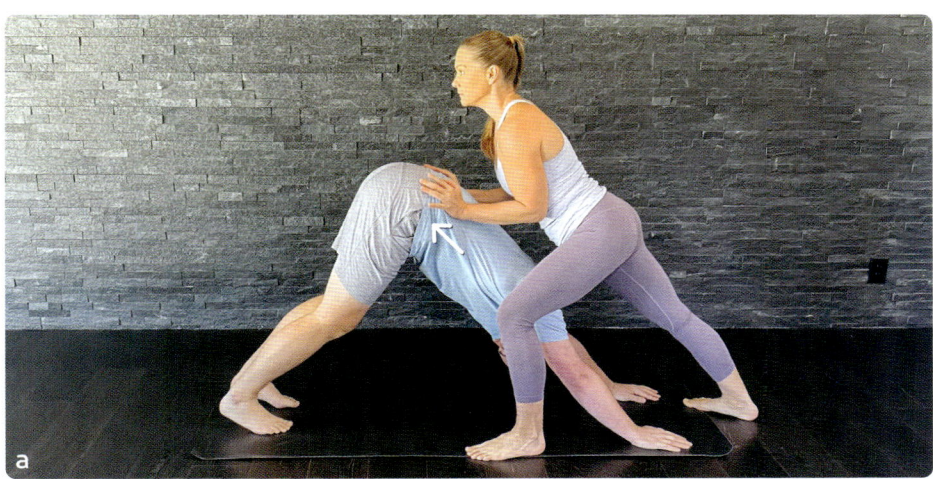

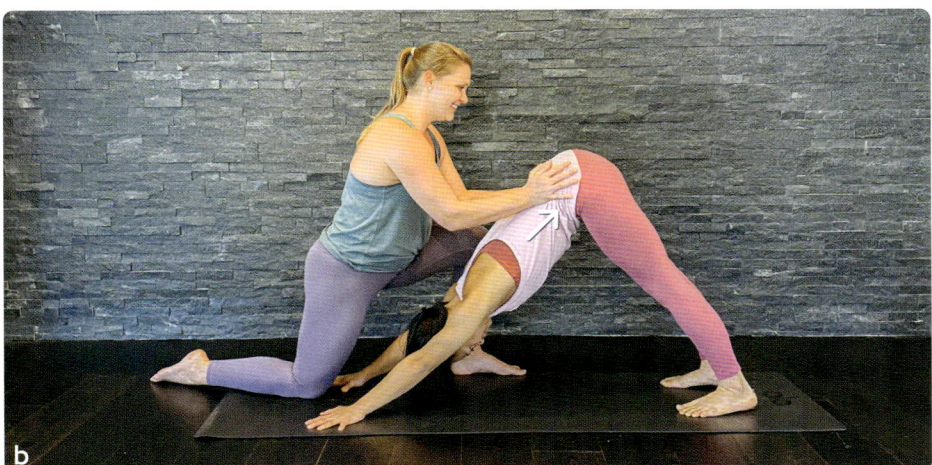

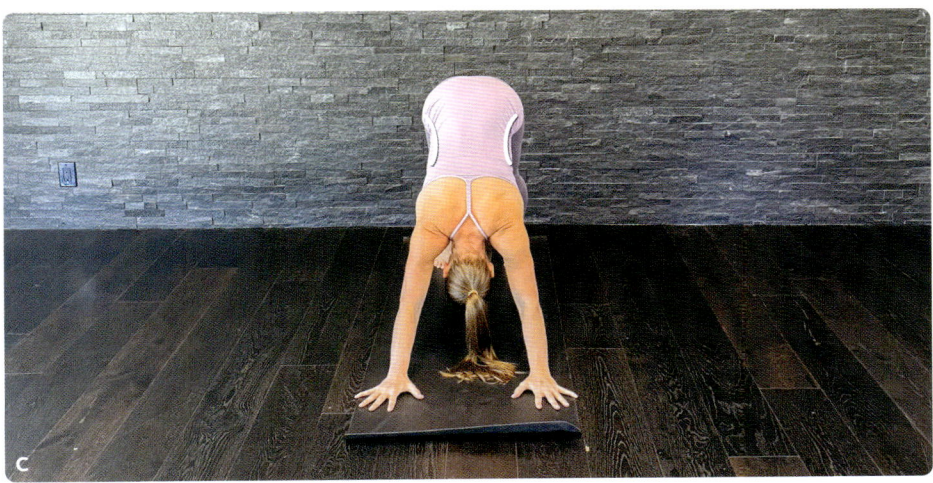

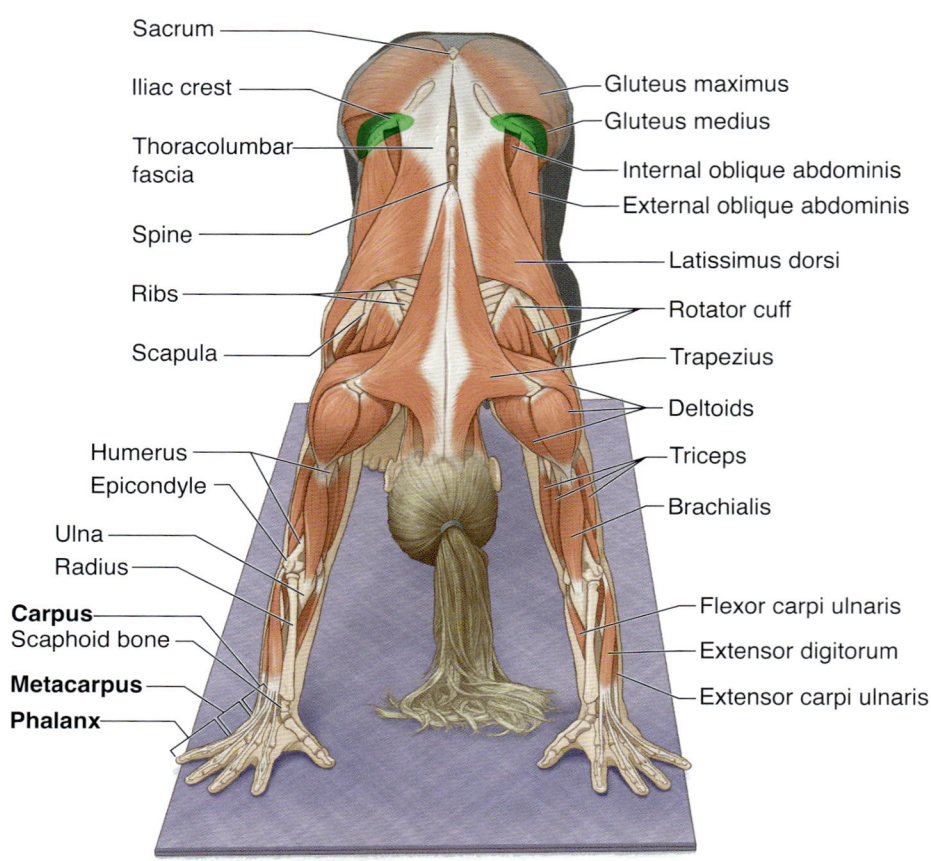

Sacrum

Iliac crest

Thoracolumbar fascia

Spine

Ribs

Scapula

Humerus

Epicondyle

Ulna

Radius

Carpus

Scaphoid bone

Metacarpus

Phalanx

Gluteus maximus

Gluteus medius

Internal oblique abdominis

External oblique abdominis

Latissimus dorsi

Rotator cuff

Trapezius

Deltoids

Triceps

Brachialis

Flexor carpi ulnaris

Extensor digitorum

Extensor carpi ulnaris

■ Stretch placement

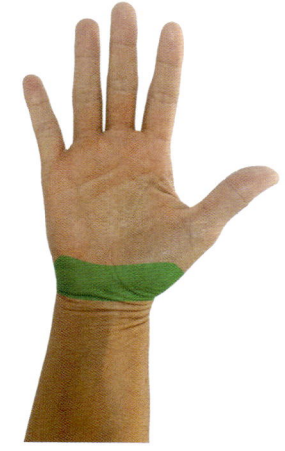

Stretch tool

STUDENT ALIGNMENT

Adho Mukha Svanasana: Downward Dog Pose

The hands are shoulder-width apart or slightly wider.

The feet are hip-width apart or wider, not to exceed the width of the mat.

The chest presses back toward the thighs.

The spine is straight from the crown of the head to the tailbone when viewed from the side.

The tailbone and hips tilt directly up or toward the ceiling.

The knees may be straight or slightly bent.

Purpose

This assist provides the student with greater ease by taking some weight off the wrists and shoulders in this inverted, arm-balancing pose. The student also receives greater stretch along the lateral sides (outside) of the torso, up through the outer shoulder region.

Stance

Variation A: Warrior I for Students Your Own Height or Taller

Using a comfortable variation of warrior I, place your dominant leg between your student's hands and root your heel. Your back leg will line up with your student's midline (the center of their body). Depending on your height, your back foot might be ahead of their hands, but it is still centered between them.

- Step your front (nondominant) leg so that the foot is approximately aligned with your student's chest. The front leg is close to your student's body, just a couple of inches from their torso.

- Square your hips toward your student. Your upper arms and elbows hug your ribs.

Variation B: Low Lunge for Students Shorter Than Your Height

Variation B uses the same basic alignment as variation A. However, you'll start by placing your front foot first. Set your front foot in alignment with your student's chest. Then, drop your back knee between your student's hands, aligning it with the midline of their body and squaring your hips toward your student.

You won't be able to hug your elbows and upper arms to your ribs, but by still hugging your elbows in, you can distribute the strength from the legs to the arms.

Anchor Placement: Provided by the Student

The rooting action of the hands in this arm-balancing pose provides the anchor for the assist.

Stretch Tool: Heel of Both Hands

Whether in variation A or B, the stretch tool and placement will be the same. Angle your wrists so that your fingers point toward 10 o'clock and 2 o'clock. Extend the wrists, drawing your fingers back toward you so that the heel of your hand is most prominent (like signaling "stop").

Stretch Placement: Iliac Crest (Top Ridge of Ilium Bones)

Take a moment to observe your student's torso in downward-facing dog. Regardless of your student's anatomical sex or body composition, everyone has a slight indentation at their true waist (as shown in image c). The true waist is the space or indentation between the ribs and the ilium bones of the pelvis. This is where you want to place your hands to apply the stretch placement.

The handholds are at the iliac crest, the top ridge of the ilium bones, at the sides of the waist. Visually find the true waist. With the heel of your hands, "scoop" into their true waist at the sides of their body and hook the heel of your hand on the top of the ilium bones. Think of the heels of your hands scooping up the ilium bones.

Follow the Lines

The lines run from your student's hands to their tailbone and mimic the lifting "up and back" actions of the pose. This is why we do not push directly toward the back of the mat or the back of the room when giving this assist. The student will feel as though you are lengthening their spine and lifting the weight of their body up, albeit slightly, out of their hands. Using the strength of your legs, press up and back toward the student's tailbone. Another way of thinking of it is to press toward where the wall meets the ceiling. You know you have it right if the student feels the weight on their hands decrease and their spine grow long without adding any pressure to their heels.

Myofascial Region

This assist involves all the myofascia along the entire torso, especially the thoracolumbar fascia at the lower back and the abdominal obliques at the sides of the core. Students may also feel a heightened stretch around their shoulder joints in most of the rotator cuff muscles, the teres major, and the latissimus dorsi.

General Precautions

If you press toward the back of the room or the back of the student's mat, this assist will not feel good to the student. Pushing straight back applies pressure to the hamstrings (backs of the thighs) and feels as though you are applying more load on the student rather than providing more space in the pose.

Common Misalignments

Generally, most people can receive this assist because it takes pressure off the hands, reduces the load on the shoulders, and lengthens the spine. If a student has very tight hamstrings, resulting in a rounded lower back, provide verbal adjustments before offering the assist. Have the student widen their feet, bend their knees, and tilt their tailbone to the sky. Provide the assist only if or when the student can flatten their lower back. If you are applying directional pressure up toward the student's tailbone, the pressure in the hamstrings will be minimal.

   If a student cannot find a straight spine in downward dog, you should not provide the assist. Also, as always, if the student looks like they're struggling in the pose, offer an adjustment instead.

Troubleshooting

Many teachers approach the stretch placement from the back as if placing their hands on the student's low back. The tissue here (the thoracolumbar fascia) is very dense and difficult to create a handhold with. Instead, approach the stretch placement from the sides of the torso, where you see the indentation of the true waist.

   Use the warrior I stance only on students who are about your height or taller, and use low-lunge stance only on students who are shorter than you. You can double-check a student's height by standing next to your student in downward dog. If their hips in downward dog are close to the height of your hips or higher, the student is about your height or taller. If their hips are lower than the height of your hips, they are shorter than you. Use either stance according to the height of your student.

   If a student is new to your class, they may think that you are trying to adjust or fix their downward dog by giving this assist. In this case, the student will start to walk their hands back toward their feet, assuming that you are trying to get them to shorten their dog. In this scenario, ask your student to firmly root their hands so that you can offer lengthening of the spine. If the student has already walked the hands back to the feet too much, they won't feel a stretch along the torso. Instead, guide them to walk their hands back out to their normal position before applying the assist. This happens so frequently that if I'm unfamiliar with the student, I will lean down and say, "Root your hands for me," and then offer the assist.

Remember to use your legs! Too many teachers try to use their arms in this assist, which can cause problems for both the teacher and the student. You know you are using your legs if your arms feel little to no effort. It will feel as though you are scooping the student's pelvis up and pressing through your legs to lift and lengthen the student's hips up and back.

Be sure to be fully in your student's space. Many teachers are afraid to step into a student's space. Unfortunately, if you are not properly aligned with your student, you can push them into misalignment. Some teachers new to this assist will press at a side angle, forcing the student's spine to become crooked by pressing the hips unevenly. This does not feel good to the student. Step into your student's space, square your hips to their hips, and press evenly with both hands, driving from the legs in an up-and-back direction toward the student's tailbone.

You may sometimes find that you lift a student up off their hands. If this happens, stop the assist, ask them to anchor their hands, and then come into the assist slower and with less pressure. Offer only enough pressure that you can feel the myofascia of the torso lengthen while the student keeps their hands rooted.

PUTTING IT ALL TOGETHER

Variation A: Student Is Taller

- Place your back foot between your student's hands at the top of their mat. Depending on your height, you may be on or off the student's mat.

- With your front foot, step into warrior I stance, roughly aligning your foot with the student's chest and ensuring your front leg is close to their body. Square your hips toward the student's body.

Variation B: Student Is Shorter

- Place your front foot first, roughly aligning your foot with the student's chest and ensuring your leg is close to their body.

- Bend your back knee and mindfully place it between your student's hands, squaring your hips toward the student's body.

• Visually look for your student's true waist—you will see a slight indentation between their ribs and hips. This is where you should place the heels of your hands.

• Turn your hands slightly outward (like turning a doorknob), pointing your fingers roughly toward 10 o'clock and 2 o'clock. Place the heels of your hands at that slight indention at the sides of their true waist.

• The heels of your hands will hook or "scoop" the ilium (pelvic bones). If you do not feel this hook or ledge on the heel of your hand, move your hands until you do.

• For variation A, bend your elbows and tuck them in toward your body. For variation B, hug your elbows towards one another in front of your chest. If needed in either variation, step closer to the student to do this. Lock your arms in place to avoid over recruitment of the arms.

• Using your legs, bend the front knee deeper and drive off the back foot or knee. Your arms do not move or change. With a tight core, the strength of the legs will be distributed through the locked arms.

• The directional pressure of the stretch is toward the student's tailbone (upward) at about a 45-degree angle. It should feel as though you have scooped up the pelvis and are lengthening it up and back.

• The student's weight lifts from their hands a bit (without the student's hands leaving the mat), helping to provide hip-to-hand lengthening. Hold this for a few moments.

• To finish the assist, rock your weight back into your back leg to give the student their weight back very slowly. Release your hands only when you feel their tissue return to its natural resting position.

Easy-Seat Side Stretch: Hip Anchor

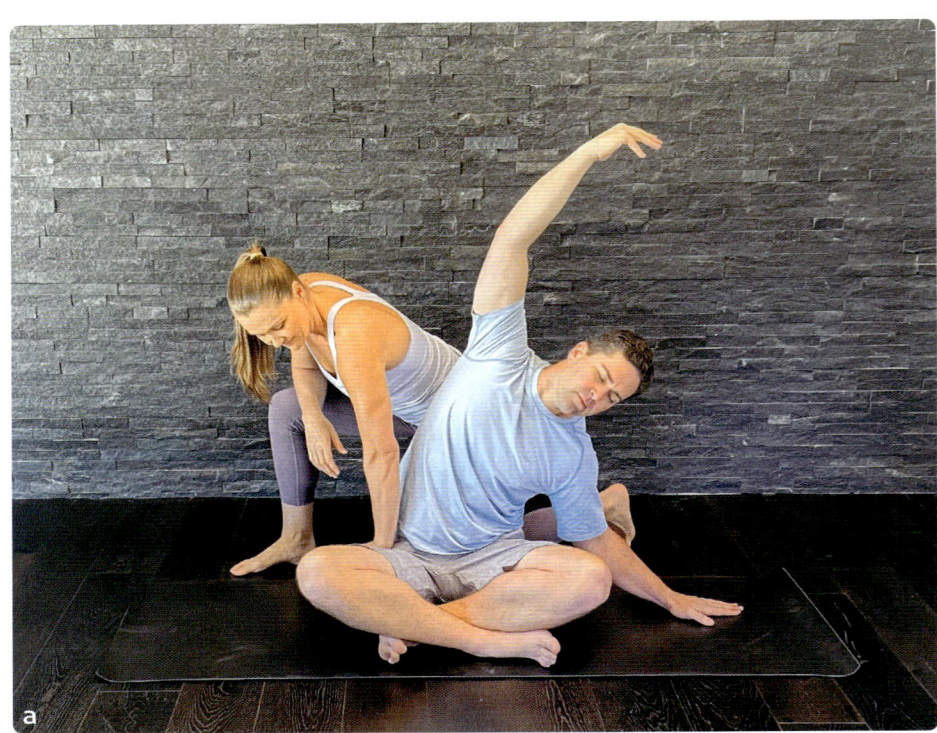

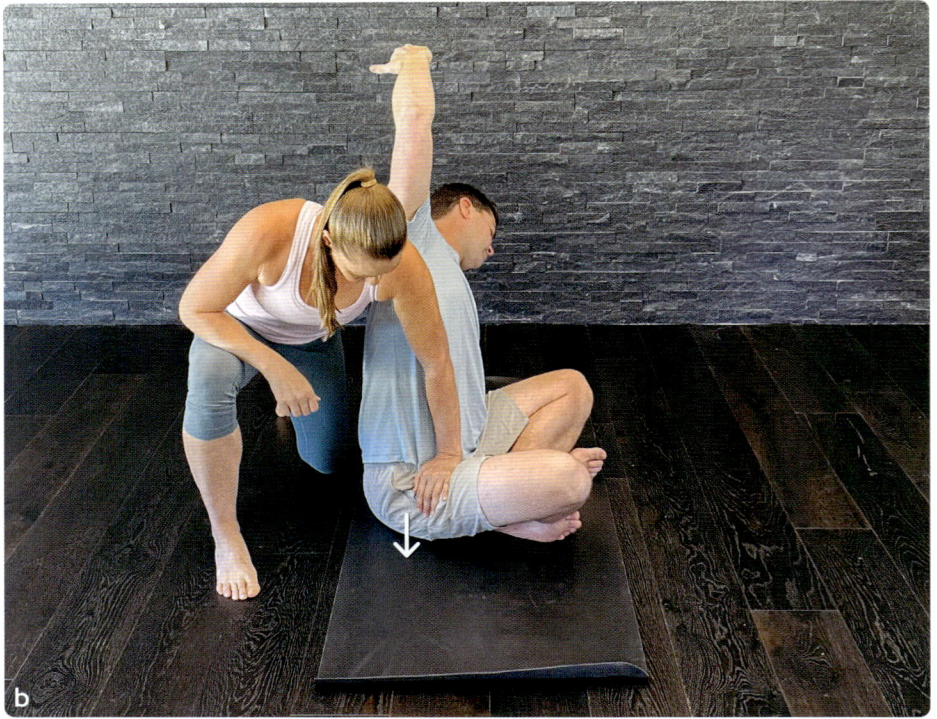

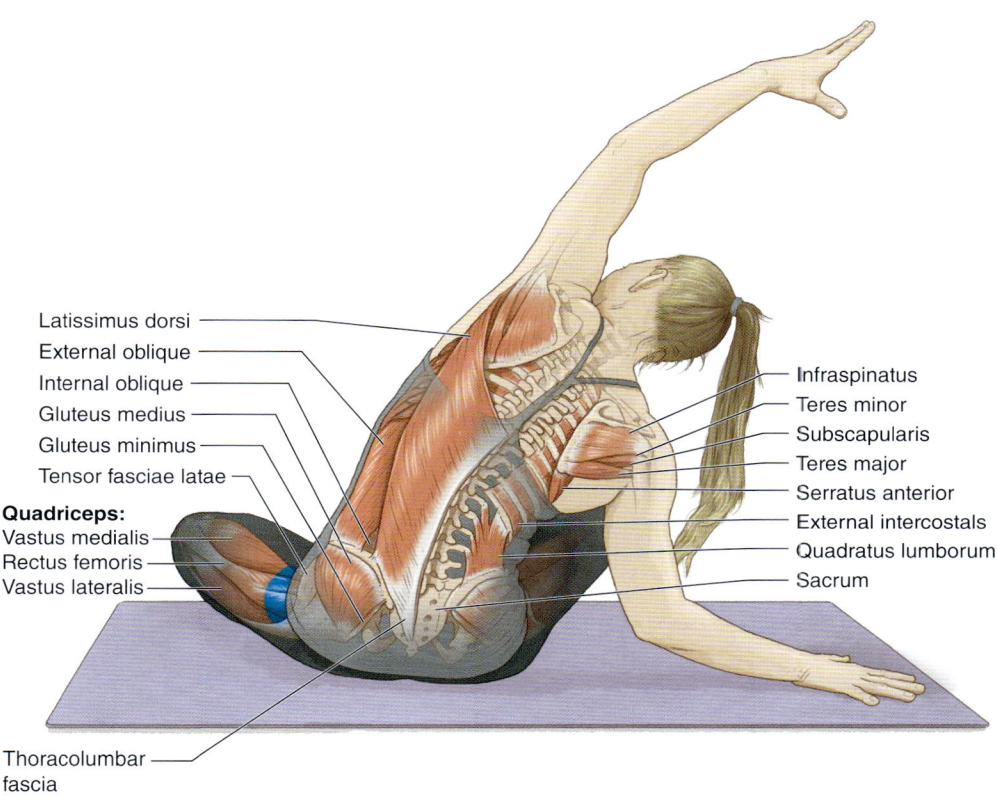

Latissimus dorsi

External oblique

Internal oblique

Gluteus medius

Gluteus minimus

Tensor fasciae latae

Quadriceps:
Vastus medialis
Rectus femoris
Vastus lateralis

Infraspinatus

Teres minor

Subscapularis

Teres major

Serratus anterior

External intercostals

Quadratus lumborum

Sacrum

Thoracolumbar
fascia

■ Anchor placement

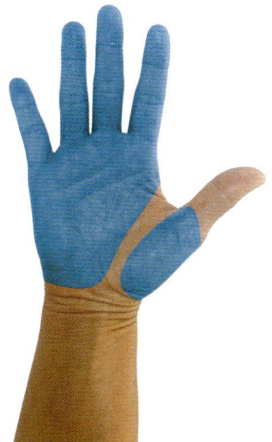

Anchor tool

Easy-Seat Side Stretch: Hip Anchor

Purpose

The action of this pose is to root the hip while lengthening up and over to one side in lateral flexion. It's common for the hip opposite the side the student is leaning toward to lift. This assist aims to assist the anchoring of this hip, which subsequently provides greater stretch along the side of the torso being stretched. Because only one side is stretched at a time, assist both sides.

Stance

Low Lunge

Alternative: Warrior I

Stand behind the student and angle your low lunge to align with the thigh you're assisting. If you are anchoring their right leg, your right leg will be forward. If you are anchoring their left leg, your left leg will be forward.

Align the shoulder of the anchor arm over your student's hip, where you will be making the anchor placement. Stack your shoulder directly over your wrist and straighten your arm to offer the anchor in this assist.

Bring your chest forward to stack your shoulder over your anchor hand. Take your opposite arm, the stretch arm, and rest your forearm on your front thigh. This will support your lower back and spine as you lean over your student to apply directional pressure.

Anchor Tool: Entire Palmar Surface of Hand

Turn your palm downward and angle your hand inward so your fingers point away from the midline of your student's body and back toward you. Allow your fingers to lightly rest against the student's thigh without grabbing or clenching their tissue.

Anchor Placement: Proximal Thigh or Upper Quadriceps

Place the thumb side of your palm high on the thigh nearest the outer hip crease. Contact the top of the thigh toward the back of the student's body or nearest you. The student's hips are open (abducted and externally rotated) in this pose, so the upper outer thigh provides plenty of soft tissue for a secure handhold.

Stretch Placement: Provided by the Student

The student creates the stretch by leaning to the side in lateral flexion. Simply applying the anchor will increase the stretch felt in the lateral torso in this pose. If they choose, they can lengthen through their fingertips to heighten the stretch with this assist.

Follow the Lines

The actions of this pose are to root the hip while lifting and lengthening through the fingertips as the torso leans to the side in lateral flexion. The assist mimics the rooting action by providing directional pressure toward the floor. The lines of stretch run from the hip to the fingertips of the arm that is extending up and over. When you anchor the hip further, the student will feel added stretch along this lateral line of the torso.

Myofascial Region

Stretch is along the lateral torso and shoulder girdle. Stretched myofascia includes the abdominal obliques, transversus abdominis, quadratus lumborum, latissimus dorsi, intercostal muscles, serratus anterior, infraspinatus, teres minor and major, and subscapularis. Compression is applied to the proximal quadriceps, the tensor fascia latae, and the gluteus medius and minimus at the outer hip crease.

General Precautions

Only offer this assist to a student who is seated on the floor or on a wide prop that mimics the floor, such as a blanket or bolster. Avoid offering this assist to a student seated on a block or any other prop that doesn't support the thighs along with the hips.

If a student is on a bolster, the bounds of their tissues will be harder to feel because their support is soft. When offering the assist to a student on a soft support, such as a bolster, think about offering just enough pressure in the anchor to resist their lateral flexion; you're offering just enough to feel the tissues pull back a little and become taut.

As with all assists, don't offer this assist to anyone with a known injury to areas the assist affects. In this case, it would primarily be the hip. This pose offers a deep oblique stretch, though, so you should also avoid providing the assist to students with abdominal injuries, such as tears or hernias.

This assist may not be appropriate to use in trauma-informed yoga settings.

Common Misalignments

The most common misalignment seen in this pose is when the student rotates their torso forward as they laterally bend. In this misaligned pose, it will look like the line from the hip to the hand is running at a diagonal towards the opposite knee rather than hand and shoulders stacked directly over the hips. A gentle adjustment to rotate the student's ribs slightly into alignment before offering the assist is an option. However, if they cannot align themselves from hip to shoulder, do not offer the assist.

If a student is not on a prop and their spine looks significantly rounded or flexed as they laterally bend, provide an adjustment in the form of a prop to sit on. Do not provide this assist for students with rounded spines.

Troubleshooting

Be mindful to leave the student's space before you guide the student or class toward the other side. The student may be deep in their practice and accidentally strike you with their arm as they come back to neutral or switch sides.

I recommend inviting students to switch the leg in front when switching sides through the arms. Students often choose a dominant leg to place in front of the other. By switching legs when switching sides, you're challenging both hips. This also helps the assist to support both legs evenly. Ideally, when doing this, you'd be assisting the hip and leg that are placed behind the other, although you can assist either leg, regardless of whether it's placed in front of or behind the other.

PUTTING IT ALL TOGETHER

- Find a low-lunge stance behind your student and angle your stance to mirror the student's thigh you'll be assisting. If assisting the right thigh, your right leg will be forward.
- Before dropping your back knee, ensure that the shoulder of your back arm lines up with the student's hip.
- Lean forward and place your front forearm, the forearm of the stretch hand, on your front thigh.
- Using your back hand, the anchor hand, position your arm and wrist so that your fingers point back toward you and away from the student.
- Using the palm of your anchor hand, place the thumb side of your palm high on the thigh, nearest the outer hip crease.
- Lean forward onto your stretch forearm and front thigh to shift the weight of your upper body forward.
- Stack your anchor shoulder over the wrist. Straighten your elbow and apply pressure directly downward toward the floor.
- Feel for the bounds of your student's tissues. This is an anchor placement only, so you will likely feel the bounds quickly and without much pressure.
- Hold the assist for a few moments. Slowly begin to release the anchor, ensuring your student's balance is stable before releasing your hand and stepping out of your student's space.
- Exit the student's space before guiding the student out of the pose.

Supine Twist: Spinal Lengthening

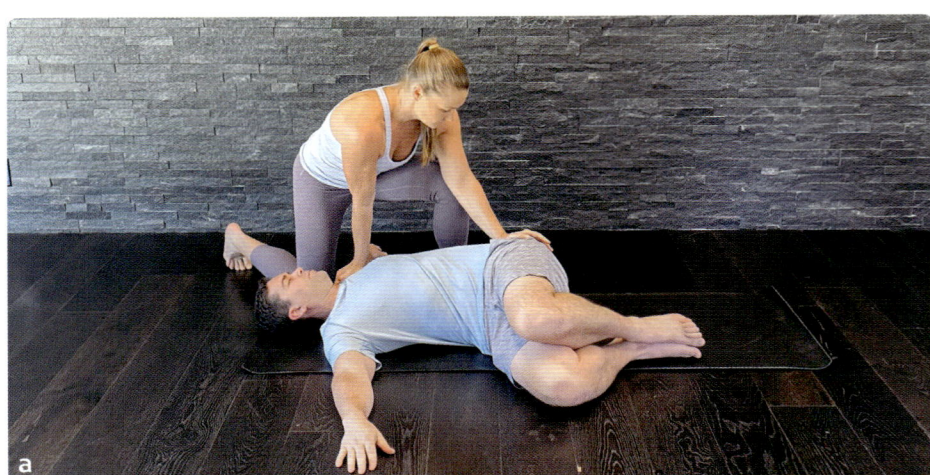

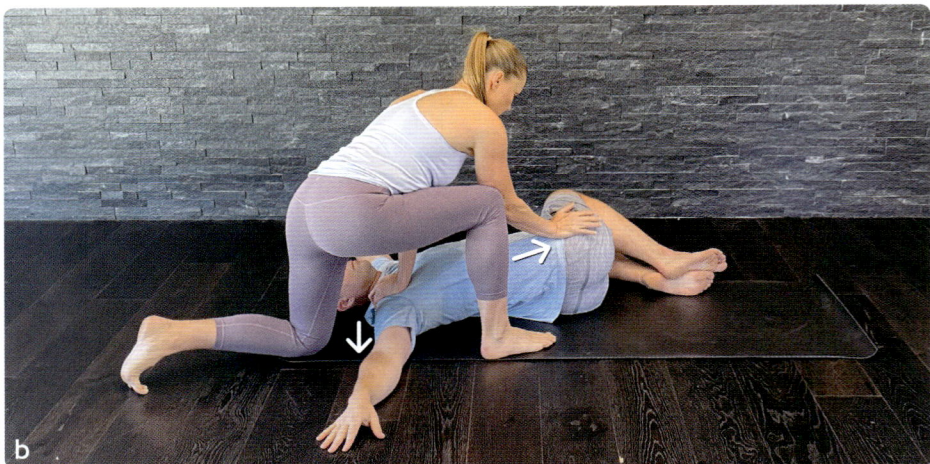

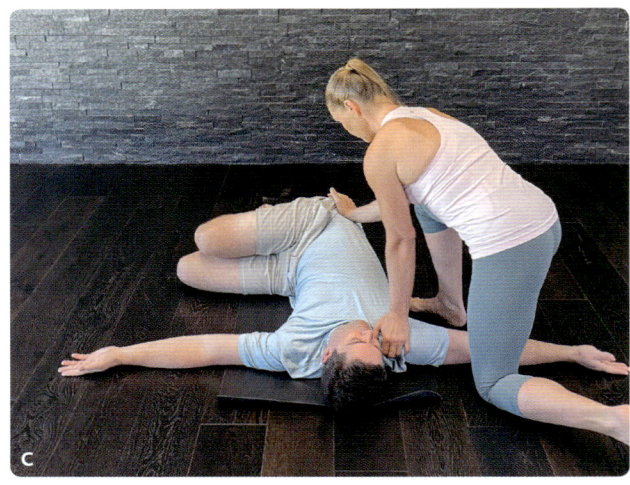

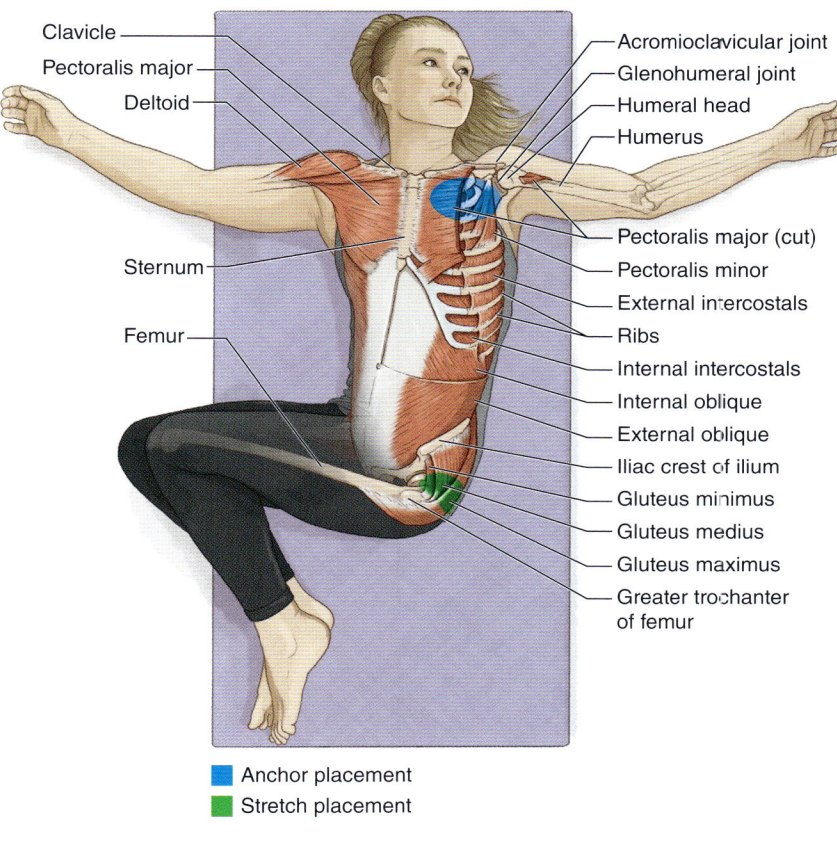

Clavicle
Pectoralis major
Deltoid
Sternum
Femur

Acromioclavicular joint
Glenohumeral joint
Humeral head
Humerus
Pectoralis major (cut)
Pectoralis minor
External intercostals
Ribs
Internal intercostals
Internal oblique
External oblique
Iliac crest of ilium
Gluteus minimus
Gluteus medius
Gluteus maximus
Greater trochanter of femur

■ Anchor placement
■ Stretch placement

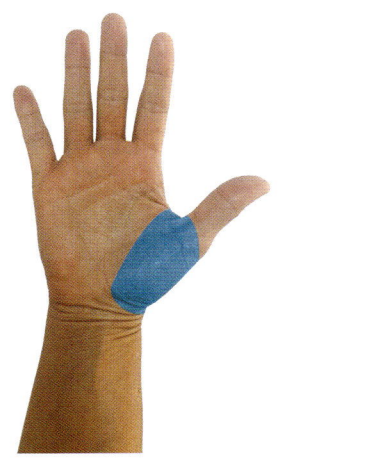

Anchor tool

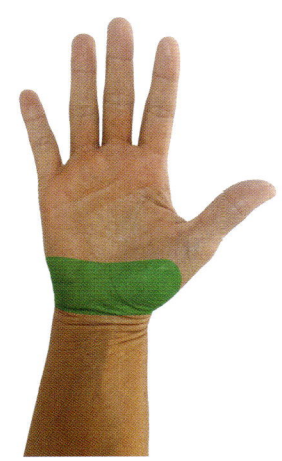

Stretch tool

> ## STUDENT ALIGNMENT
>
> ### Supta Matsyendrasana: Supine Twist Pose
>
> Both shoulders root to the earth, with the arms open to cactus or *T*.
>
> The knees are bent and resting on one side of the body on either the mat or a prop.
>
> The knees roughly align with the height of the hips or higher.
>
> The student appears still and comfortable in the pose.

Purpose

This assist accentuates the line of stretch felt between the hip and the shoulder. Avoid pushing the student's hips deeper into the twist. When you anchor the student's shoulder, they will feel a greater sense of grounding in this passive pose as well. Because one side is stretched at a time, you should assist both sides. This assist can be provided to students in variations of supine twist where both knees are bent or in variations with the bottom leg straight.

Stance

Low Lunge

If your student is twisted with the knees to the left, your right foot will be forward. If your student is twisted with the knees to the right, your left foot will be forward. Place your back knee above and near your student's shoulder. Note that you are stepping over the student's outstretched arm.

The anchor arm will remain straight, with the shoulder stacked over the wrist. The stretch arm will stack the elbow directly in front of the kneecap to use the strength of the legs to apply directional pressure.

Anchor Tool: Thenar Eminence (Base of Thumb)

Using the hand of your back arm, turn your palm downward and angle your wrist outward so that your fingers point away from the student's chest. The thenar eminence, or the base of the thumb, will apply the pressure. To make the assist feel soft rather than rigid, allow the rest of your hand to rest lightly on the student's shoulder.

See Bound-Angle Chest Press, page 196, for more information on this portion of the assist.

Anchor Placement: Pectoralis Major, Upper and Outer Chest

There is a depression that feels like a soft semicircle of tissue on the chest that borders the humeral head. Position the base of your thumb in this soft semicircle so that you place pressure on the chest rather than the shoulder (glenohumeral) joint. With the base of the thumb at this soft semicircle of tissue, you can lightly cup the humeral head with the rest of your hand and wrap your fingers around the top of the shoulder without applying pressure to the shoulder specifically.

As a reminder, always place the anchor first and release it last.

See Bound-Angle Chest Press, page 196, for more information on this portion of the assist.

Stretch Tool: Heel of Hand

Extend your wrist and lift your fingers lightly to bring the heel of the hand forward (like signaling "stop"). Be mindful to keep your hand soft when using the heel of your hand. If you extend or lift your fingers too much, it'll make your palm rigid. Instead, lift your fingers only enough to keep from laying them on your student's hip.

Stretch Placement: Gluteus Medius and Minimus, Outer Hip

Place your stretch hand just above the greater trochanter of the femur (outer hip bone) on the gluteus medius and minimus muscles, which are superior to (above) the greater trochanter.

Do not place the stretch hand on the hip crease; instead, visually find the hip crease and imagine a line extending outward toward the outer hip. The greater trochanter and the two gluteus muscles are on the lateral (outer) hip.

At the outer hip, you will notice a bony mound (greater trochanter) indicating where to place your palm. Just above this bony landmark are the muscles and soft tissues where you will apply pressure with the heel of your hand. You know you have it right if it feels like you have hooked the hip bone with the heel of your hand.

Follow the Lines

You are following the line of the torso and not the line of the twist. You should feel a sense of elongating the torso from the shoulder to the hip rather than assisting the student deeper into rotation.

Place the anchor first by applying pressure directly downward. This mimics the action of the pose, in which the student aims to keep the shoulder rooted to the mat. While keeping consistent pressure on the anchor, use the heel of your hand to hook into the soft tissue of the outer hip. Slowly sink your hips and bend into your front knee. Bending your front knee will transmit the strength of the legs through the elbow and forearm and into the stretch hand. The direction of the stretch application follows the line of the student's torso, which means you're pressing toward the student's tailbone. Think about lengthening the line between your anchor and stretch hands. Do not press the student's hips toward the floor or toward the student's knees; press in the direction in which the tailbone is pointed. You can also think of this directional pressure as pressing toward the feet.

Myofascial Region

This assist stretches all the myofascia along the lateral torso, especially the thoracolumbar fascia, quadratus lumborum, abdominal obliques, intercostal muscles, and applies compression to the pectoralis major and minor. This assist unilaterally lengthens the torso.

General Precautions

Avoid pushing a student's hips deeper into rotation. Doing so creates a greater risk of injuring the lumbar spine and the hips. When offering this assist, align your body to be parallel with the student's torso so that when you apply the stretch application, you will feel a sense of lengthening the torso rather than pushing the student into a deeper rotation.

The core is enveloped in thick fascia both anteriorly (in the abdominal wall) and posteriorly (in the low back). The abdominal aponeurosis and the thoracolumbar fascia are dense with collagen, and although these fascial structures stretch more in spinal extension and flexion, the lateral side body stretching still affects both simultaneously, particularly at their lateral attachments. Some people can feel extremely flexible and mobile in their tissues here, whereas others can feel extremely dense. Trust that as soon as you feel the tissues become taut, that's enough pressure; hold that bound, and don't press past it.

Some people have remarkably flexible pelvises that tilt easily. When you apply the directional pressure with the stretch hand, their pelvis tilts and seems to move significantly. When you encounter a student with a pelvis like this, back off on your stretch pressure and emphasize your anchor pressure instead. If the student's pelvis dramatically shifts, don't offer more directional pressure; rather, back off and ensure their pelvis remains in its initial resting position.

Avoid offering this assist to anyone with hip injuries or conditions.

Common Misalignments

It can be difficult to assist a student in this shape if they do not have their knees in alignment with their hips because the soft ledge of gluteus tissue above the greater trochanter won't be prominent. It's difficult to have a secure handhold without the handhold being prominent. If a student has taken their twist with their knees only slightly bent rather than bent and lifted to about the height of the hips, there will be little tissue to hold on to at the hip. Skip this student and find another who provides a better handhold for the stretch placement.

If the student's shoulder opposite the knees is lifted, do not offer this assist. The student is already getting a strong stretch from the hip to the shoulder; they don't need more stretch.

Troubleshooting

After you have placed your hand on the student's hip, don't be afraid to move it if you do not have a good handhold. You do not want to apply directional pressure and suddenly slip off the student's hip. If I begin pressure at the stretch placement and recognize that my handhold isn't as secure as I'd like, I'll back off the pressure and press the heel of my hand into their hip (similar to gently palpating for the correct spot) until I find a secure handhold, then apply directional pressure again. Note that while I'm finding this new stretch placement, I'm still maintaining the anchor pressure at the chest.

Though it may seem like the hip crease would be a good handhold, it is not. If you apply pressure to the hip crease, this will only press the student's thigh away.

Supine Twist: Spinal Lengthening

Be sure you are comfortable when giving this assist. If you do not have a good handhold on the student's hip, you risk slipping off the student's body and falling on top of them. If you feel like you are reaching, step farther into their space. If you sense that your arms are doing all the work, remember to place the elbow in front of the knee so that the legs can deliver the strength of the assist. Finally, if your back knee is sensitive in the low-lunge position, do not hesitate to place your knee on your student's mat near their head or grab a blanket to slide beneath you.

Depending on your stature and that of your student, it can sometimes feel like you're putting your sensitive areas too close to the student's head. In these instances, rely on your anchor arm as a barrier, and angle your hips away from their face.

PUTTING IT ALL TOGETHER

- Place your back knee above and near the student's shoulder opposite the direction in which they are twisted. If they are twisted to the right, your right knee will be down. If they are twisted to the left, your left knee will be down.

- Step the opposite foot over their outstretched arm, placing it roughly in alignment with their midback. Find the low-lunge stance, ensuring your legs and hips mirror or are parallel to the line of the student's spine.

- Anchor with your back arm, using the base of your thumb to create a chest press. Stack your shoulder over your wrist, keep your arm straight, and press directly toward the floor. Maintain this anchor pressure until the end of the assist.

- Visually find the mound of tissue and bone at the student's outer hip. Place your palm on this mound, and then sink the heel of your hand into the tissues directly above it. You should feel the heel of your hand hook into the soft ledge of tissue directly above the hip bone.

- Before applying directional pressure at the hip, move your front foot and place your kneecap directly behind your elbow. It should look like a straight line from the hip to the knee to the hand.

- Maintaining directional pressure in the anchor hand directly downward, sink your hips and bend into your front knee, applying directional pressure to the stretch hand.

- Moving slowly, direct the line of stretch toward the student's tailbone or feet and not toward their knees. Stop and hold when you feel a tightening of the tissues on their lateral torso (the side of the body).

- Hold the stretch for a few moments. Finish the assist by rocking your hips back slowly until the student's tissues return to their natural resting position. Release the anchor hand last.

Deer Pose: Spinal Lengthening

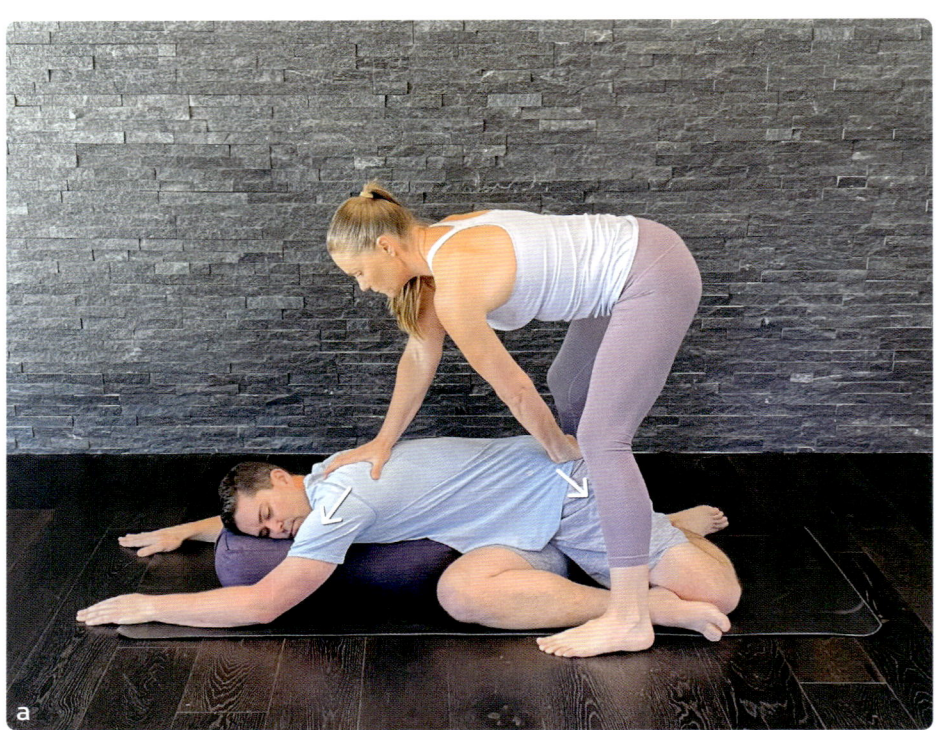

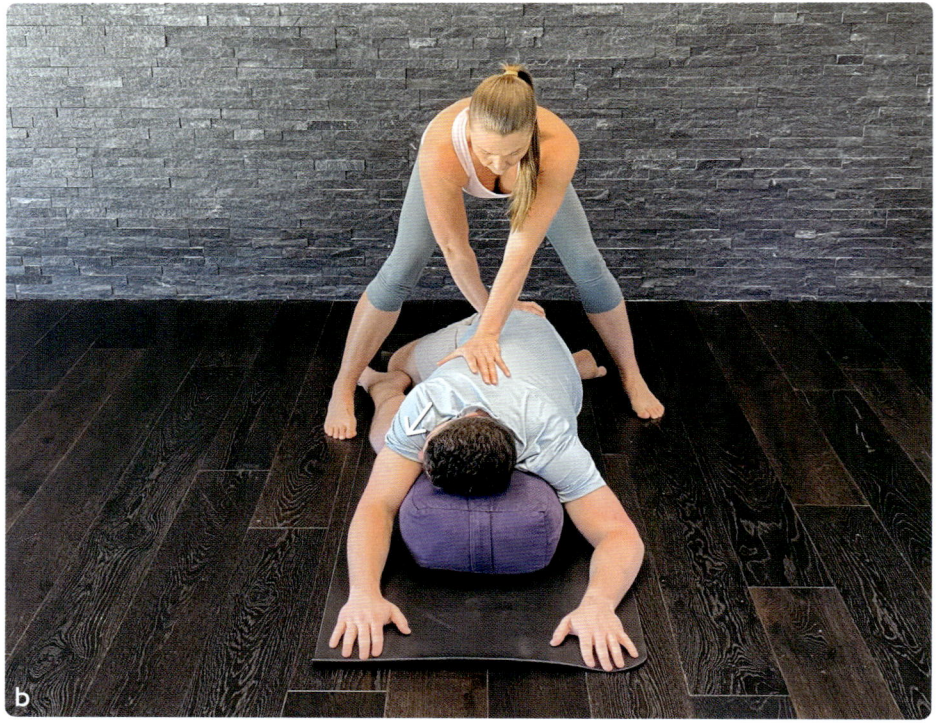

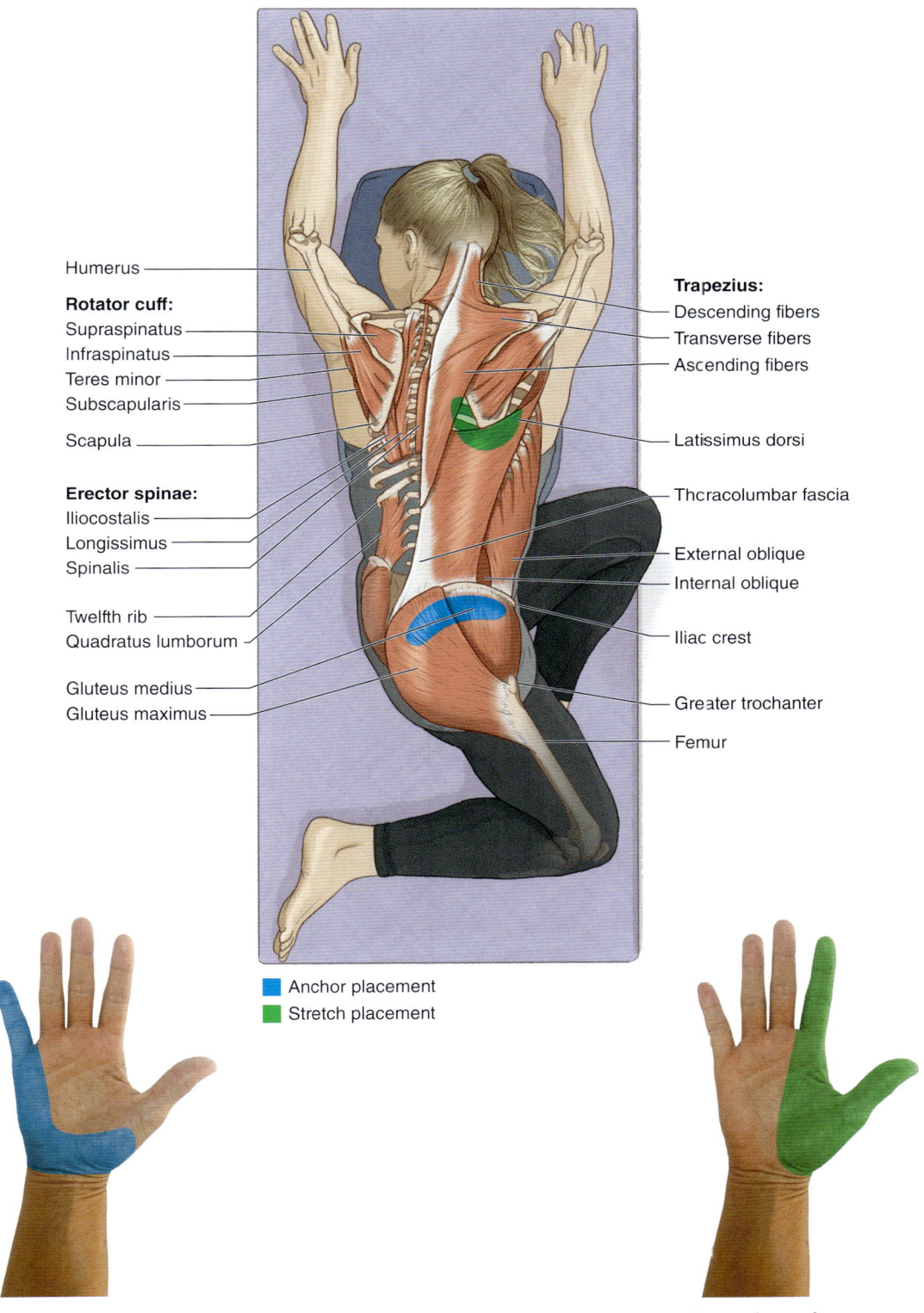

Humerus

Rotator cuff:
Supraspinatus
Infraspinatus
Teres minor
Subscapularis

Scapula

Erector spinae:
Iliocostalis
Longissimus
Spinalis

Twelfth rib
Quadratus lumborum

Gluteus medius
Gluteus maximus

Trapezius:
Descending fibers
Transverse fibers
Ascending fibers

Latissimus dorsi

Thoracolumbar fascia

External oblique
Internal oblique

Iliac crest

Greater trochanter

Femur

■ Anchor placement
■ Stretch placement

Anchor tool

Stretch tool

STUDENT ALIGNMENT

Mrigasana: Deer Pose

The legs are either scissored or stacked one on top of the other.

The torso is fully supported by a bolster running parallel to the student's spine.

Both shoulders are squared toward the bolster.

The arms extend toward the top of the mat; the elbows are ahead of the shoulders.

The head is rotated either toward or away from the knees, based on the student's comfort.

Purpose

Deer pose is a prone twist that emphasizes a unilateral stretch along the back of the body. This assist emphasizes the line of stretch along one side of the back, from the pelvis to the shoulder. Because this pose stretches one side at a time, you should assist both sides.

Stance

High Squat

Roughly align your heels with your student's midthighs. Adjust your stance accordingly to ensure your shoulders stack over the anchor placement at the student's hip.

Your legs will help you hold the anchor. As you press the anchor hand down or toward the student's feet, bend your knees slightly and sink into your heels, drawing the weight of your body backward in the same direction as the anchor pressure.

Anchor Tool: Palm of the Hand with Prominence Toward the Hypothenar Eminence (Pinky Side of the Palm)

The shape of the tool, or how you hold your hand, will mimic the semicircle shape of the handhold. Create a cupping action with your hand, as if you are holding water in your palm. Then, turn your palm downward and angle your fingers inward so that the pinky side of your hand is pointing forward. Hook into the tissue with the pinky side of your palm while maintaining the cupping shape with your hand.

The anchor hand will be the hand that matches the same side as the student's hip you're anchoring. If you're assisting their right hip, the anchor is your right hand. If you're assisting their left hip, the anchor is your left hand. You will crisscross your arms with your anchor and stretch placements. This allows you to use more strength in your chest—namely, your pectoralis major muscles.

Anchor Placement: Gluteus Medius, Soft Tissue Inferior to the Iliac Crest

The anchor is at the posterolateral iliac crest, the pelvic bone found at the base of the spine and lower back. Look for the bony ridge of the iliac crest of the ilium and aim to contact the soft tissue just inferior to (beneath) this ridge. The pinky side of your palm will hook into the soft tissue between the iliac crest and the greater trochanter of the hip. As a result, it may feel like your palm is cupping the hip.

Stretch Tool: The Hooked Surface Between Index Finger and Thumb

The stretch tool mimics the shape of the shoulder blade. You will apply most of the pressure with the area between the index finger and the base of the thumb, although your whole hand can rest on the student's back.

Stretch Placement: Transverse and Ascending Fibers of Trapezius, Latissimus Dorsi; Soft Tissue Bordering Medial Border and Inferior Angle of the Scapula

The shoulder to assist is on the same side as the hip you're assisting; for example, if you're assisting the right hip, you'll assist the right shoulder.

Align your index finger and thumb around the medial border and inferior angle of the student's shoulder blade. Your fingers will run parallel to the medial border of the shoulder blade, and your thumb will hook the inferior angle. The placement is not on the shoulder blade but rather on the soft tissue just medial and inferior to, or just outside of, the shoulder blade.

Follow the Lines

The lines follow the latissimus dorsi muscle. Imagine a large V shape running from the sacrum and hips out toward the shoulder. You are following this diagonal line from the sacrum to the shoulder.

Apply the anchor first and maintain pressure throughout. Using more of the pinky side of your palm, press inferiorly toward the student's back knee or the feet. The direction is back toward you rather than directly downward. If you were to press directly downward, it would press the student's hips into the floor, which would not feel good. Note that the anchor is only on one hip, the hip that is stacked on top.

Sink your stretch hand into the student's tissues alongside the medial and inferior angle of the scapula. Gently press in toward the rib cage to hook into the myofascia, and then press at a diagonal toward the humeral head or outer shoulder. You can also think of it as pressing toward the student's elbow.

You are feeling for the line of stretch between your two hands, at the lateral hip or anchor and the shoulder blade or stretch placement

Myofascial Region

Stretch will occur in the thoracolumbar fascia, quadratus lumborum, spinal erectors, latissimus dorsi, and ascending trapezius. You will apply stretch compression to the latissimus dorsi and ascending trapezius. You will apply anchor compression to the glutes, specifically the gluteus medius.

General Precautions

Many people have dense lower back tissue or thoracolumbar fascia. Be mindful to listen to your hands and not apply too much pressure. The tissue should feel supple between your hands. If you feel a tightening of the tissue between your hands or a sense that the tissue is resisting, that's the boundary; do not apply more pressure. A little goes a long way in this region because it's very collagen dense.

Common Misalignments

If a student cannot rotate fully and place their chest squarely on the bolster, do not offer this assist. You may need to offer the student a block to place beneath their bolster to provide elevation and more assistance to the spinal twist. A student who cannot twist completely will usually look as though they are lying sideways with one shoulder on the bolster. This student needs an adjustment in their props rather than a Rubber Band Method® assist.

Troubleshooting

Many students will pull their elbows toward their sides in this shape, as if hugging the bolster. If you apply pressure near the shoulder blade, it will press the student's elbow into the floor. This is uncomfortable for the student and can cause the assist to move into the neck. Consider gently moving the student's arms and elbows forward a bit, or use cuing to invite them to lengthen their arms farther forward before relaxing.

The range of motion in the scapulae can vary considerably from student to student. Be sure to look for the bony landmarks of the scapula to help you identify the handhold. The scapulae are not always located close to the spine; in mobile students, they are often upwardly rotated a great deal away from the spine.

PUTTING IT ALL TOGETHER

- Step over your student and find a high-squat stance, aligning your heels with their mid- to upper thighs.

- Create the anchor with the arm that matches the same side as the hip you're assisting. Visually find the ilium or pelvic bone at the lower back. Using the pinky side of your palm, hook into the tissue just inferior to the ilium and press inferiorly toward the student's feet or back towards you.

- Maintain the pressure of the anchor by recruiting your legs. Sink into your heels and draw your body weight backward in the same direction in which you're anchoring.

- Look for the medial border (inner edge) of the shoulder blade to place your stretch hand. Using the space between your index finger and thumb on your opposite hand, sink into the tissue around the inferior angle of the scapula. Once you are hooked into the tissue, gently apply directional pressure toward the shoulder. There should be little to no movement of the scapula.

- Apply directional pressure slowly to feel for the resistance or tightening of tissue between your two hands as you apply the stretch.

- When you feel the tissues become taut or give some resistance to the stretch, pause and hold the assist for a few moments.

- To release the assist, gently back out of the stretch and then release the anchor hand last, ensuring your student's tissues have returned to their natural resting position before removing your anchor hand completely.

11
NECK AND SHOULDERS

Bound Angle or Corpse Pose: Chest Press
Corpse Pose: Neck Traction
Deer Pose: Reverse Shoulder Press

Bound Angle or Corpse Pose: Chest Press

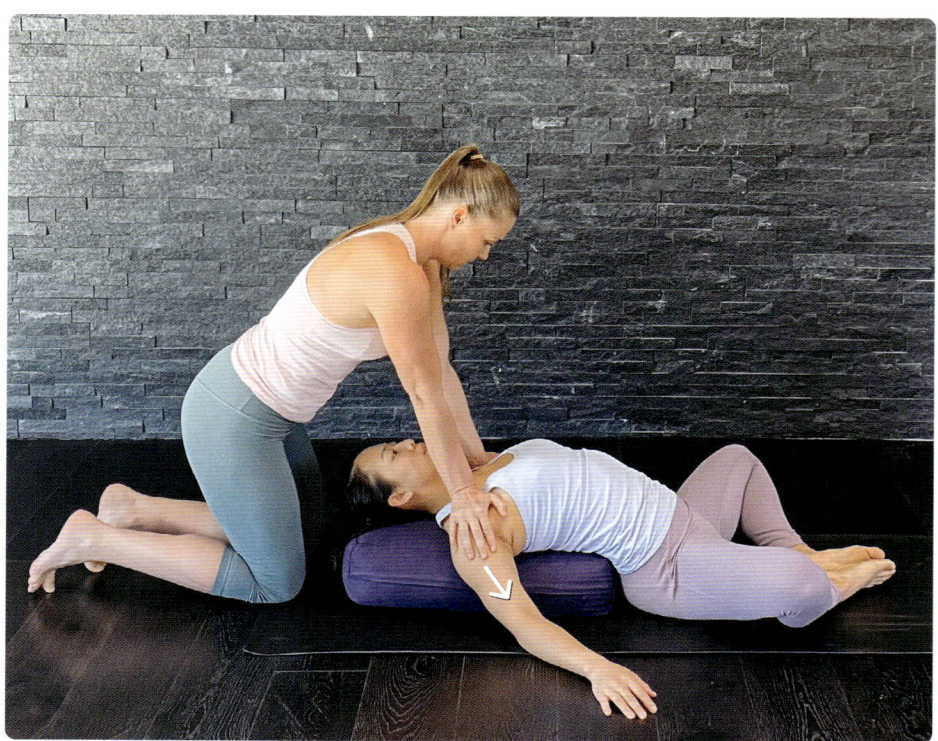

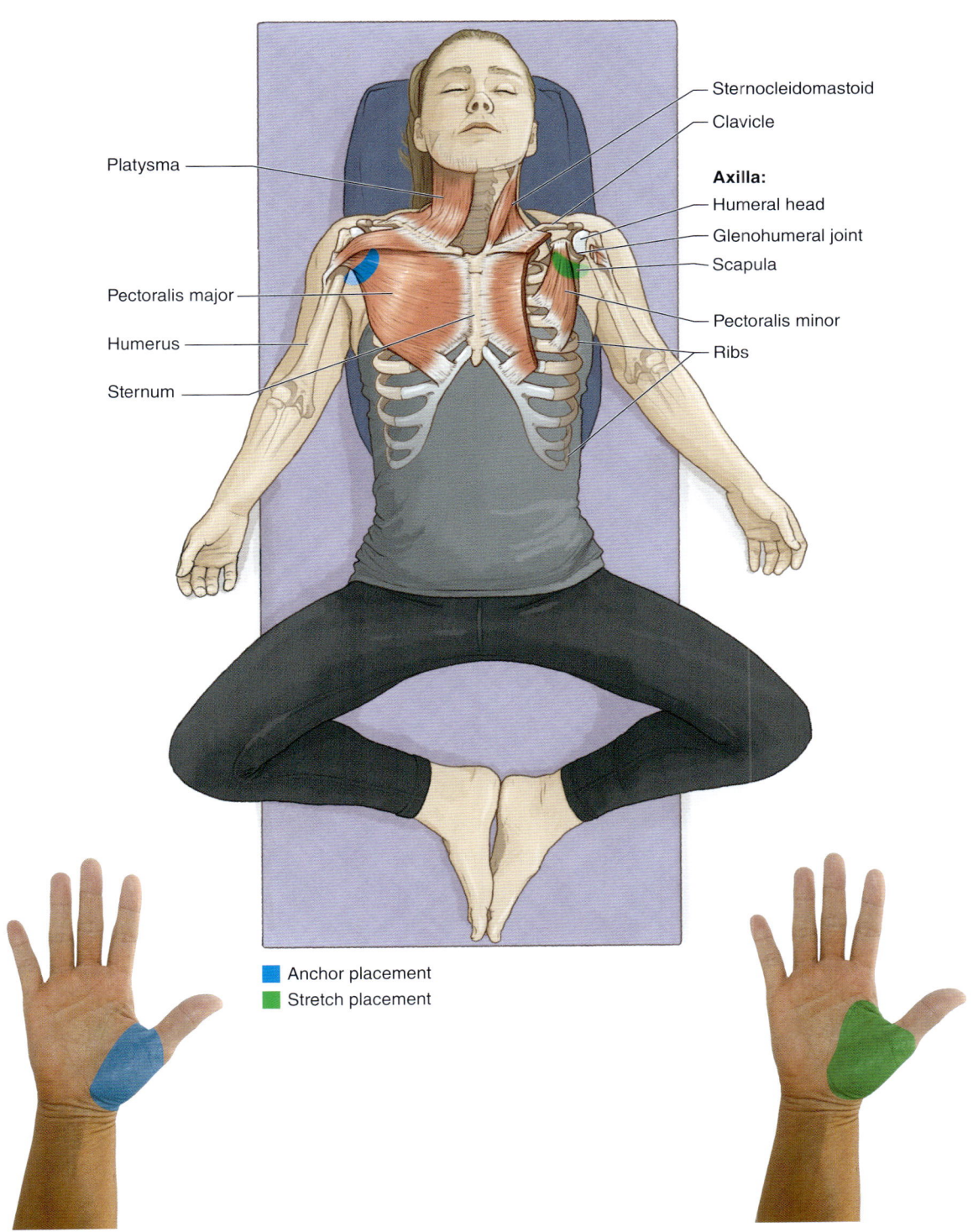

Sternocleidomastoid

Clavicle

Axilla:

Humeral head

Glenohumeral joint

Scapula

Platysma

Pectoralis minor

Pectoralis major

Ribs

Humerus

Sternum

■ Anchor placement
■ Stretch placement

Anchor tool

Stretch tool

STUDENT ALIGNMENT

Supta Baddha Konasana: Reclined Bound-Angle Pose

The soles of the feet are together. The knees are open wide, with or without the support of a prop.

The torso rests passively on a bolster supporting the full length of the torso, from the lower back to the back of the head.

The arms are open passively at the student's sides, with the back of the hands or palms resting against the mat.

The head is supported by the bolster or a low blanket.

Purpose

Supported reclined bound angle is a restorative pose that is both a chest and hip opener. By providing a chest press, the assist increases the sense of grounding and accentuates the lines of stretch across the chest. The chest press assist can also be applied in corpse pose to facilitate a gentle chest stretch and added sense of grounding.

Stance

Kneeling

Alternative: High-Squat Stance

Place your knees directly behind the student's head. When giving the assist, lift your hips to bring your shoulders directly over your wrists and the student's chest. Your arms should remain straight throughout the assist.

Anchor Tool: Thenar Eminence (Base of Thumb)

The anchor tool is identical to the stretch tool. The hands will alternate back and forth in a palpating rhythm. The hand applying pressure is the stretch; the hand providing a counterbalance or stabilization is the anchor.

Anchor Placement: Lateral Pectoralis Major, Outer Corner of the Chest Bordering the Axilla (Armpit)

See Stretch Placement.

Stretch Tool: Thenar Eminence (Base of Thumb)

Turn your palms down and angle your hands outward so your fingers point away from the student's chest and back towards you. If your fingers were the hands of a clock, they'd be pointing toward 4 o'clock and 8 o'clock.

You will use the thenar eminence, or base of the thumb, to apply the directional pressure. The rest of the palm and hand can lightly rest on the student's shoulder.

Stretch Placement: Lateral Pectoralis Major, Outer Corner of the Chest Bordering the Axilla (Armpit)

Align the thenar eminence (thumb pad) of each hand with the soft semicircle of tissue at the corners of the chest, nearest the axillae (armpits). With the thumb pad placed in this depression on the chest, you can ensure that there is no strong pressure on the shoulder (glenohumeral) joint; instead, the pressure is against the chest rather than the shoulder itself.

To find this placement, palpate your own shoulder to explore what you are looking for. Find the humeral head, the round knob at the top of your arm that we refer to as the shoulder. From this place, move your fingers an inch or two (2-5 cm) diagonally toward the center of your chest. There is a depression that feels like a soft semicircle of tissue on the chest that surrounds the humeral head. The axilla is at one end of this soft semicircle. The other end is roughly at the lateral (outside) end of your clavicle (collarbone); you will usually feel a bony protrusion here nearest the shoulder. Place the thumb pad of your hand in this soft semicircle so that you direct your pressure to the ribs rather than the shoulder joints.

With the base of the thumb at this soft semicircle of tissue, you can lightly cup the humeral head with the rest of your hand and wrap your fingers around the top of the shoulder without applying pressure to the shoulder specifically.

Follow the Lines

The lines of stretch run across the chest from shoulder to shoulder. Imagine that you are broadening or widening the chest with this assist. The directional pressure is out and down, at an angle rather than directly toward the floor.

Offer this assist with alternating pressure from side to side. As one hand applies directional pressure for the stretch placement, the opposite hand remains where it is as a counterbalance. This counterbalance acts as the anchor. Alternate your hands as you apply directional pressure back and forth, slowly, without lifting either hand from the student's body until the end of the assist.

Because this is an alternating assist, I always end by applying pressure with both of my hands simultaneously, albeit with very little pressure. This provides a pause and signals to the student that the assist is ending.

Myofascial Region

The pectoralis majors are compressed and stretched. Depending on the student, some additional stretch may be felt through the neck via the platysma and sternocleidomastoid.

General Precautions

Many people have shoulder injuries or issues, and you must take caution when offering this assist. Although this assist is to the chest and ribs, it still stretches tissues that insert into the shoulder. Be mindful to go in slowly to read the cues you receive from your student's tissues. If you apply pressure with a sense of spreading the chest apart rather than pushing down, it will feel good to the student without much pressure needed.

You may feel a pop or shift beneath your hand; let that be a signal to back off and, if need be, check in with the student on their comfort.

If a student has a lot of breast tissue, do not offer this assist. Because of the nature of breast tissue, it can move superiorly, or more toward the collarbone, when someone is lying in a supine position. This limits the space to safely place your thenar eminence against the upper ribs or chest. Without enough space at the upper chest, you risk touching breast tissue or applying pressure directly to the shoulder. You must avoid both scenarios.

This assist may not be appropriate to use in trauma-informed yoga settings.

Common Misalignments

There generally aren't misalignments with this pose. That being said, if a student is in this pose with their arms by their sides, rather than opened away from the body, or with their palms turned down, they won't feel as much of an opening across the chest. If your student has a shoulder injury or pain, avoid giving chest and shoulder assists altogether.

Troubleshooting

If you feel this assist in your lower back as you provide it, lean over your student more, ensuring you stack your shoulders over your wrists. If you are giving many chest-press assists in class, you can instead give this assist using high-squat stance.

If you are still learning how to read tissues, opt to only alternate pressure rather than pressing on both sides of the chest simultaneously. Alternating pressure is the safest way to avoid pressing too hard.

PUTTING IT ALL TOGETHER

- Drop your knees close to the student's head and find a kneeling stance.
- While standing on your knees, shift your weight over the student so that your shoulders stack over their shoulders.
- Look for the student's shoulder heads. There is a small indention on either side of the chest where the rib cage meets the shoulder. This is the soft semicircle where you place the base of your thumb.
- Turning your fingers away from the chest and toward the student's arms, place the base or pad of the thumbs in these depressions at the corners of the chest.
- Allow your palms to rest lightly on the rounded heads of the shoulders. Your fingers are welcome to rest lightly on the arms of the student, but do not grasp the tissue.
- Gently and slowly apply directional pressure into the thumb pads to one side of the chest at a time while keeping both hands on your student. The direction of the pressure is at an angle outward and downward, toward the arms.
- The opposite hand at the same location on the other side of the chest acts as a counterbalance, resisting the pressure of the stretch hand. This counterbalance is the anchor. Between your two hands, you should sense that the assist is spreading the chest.
- Alternate pressure back and forth between the two hands in a slow, rhythmic palpation. Be mindful to listen for how the tissues are stretching, and be sure to stop when you feel resistance. A little pressure often goes a long way.
- To complete the assist, gently press both sides of the chest lightly, with half the amount or less of pressure. Release both hands slowly, ensuring the student's tissues have returned to their natural resting position before removing both hands completely.

Corpse Pose: Neck Traction

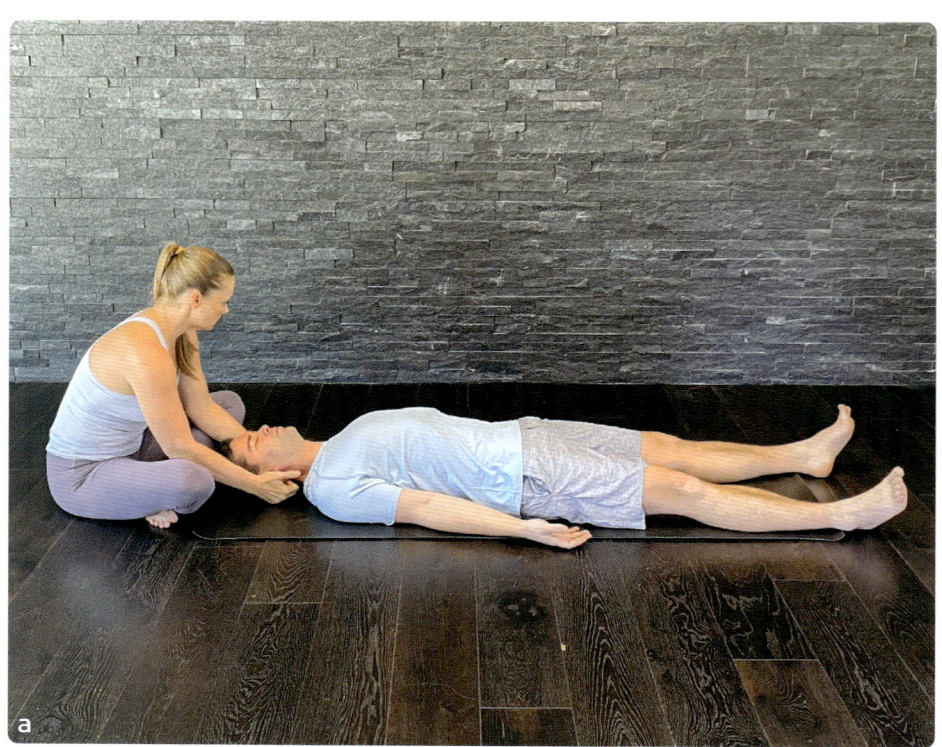

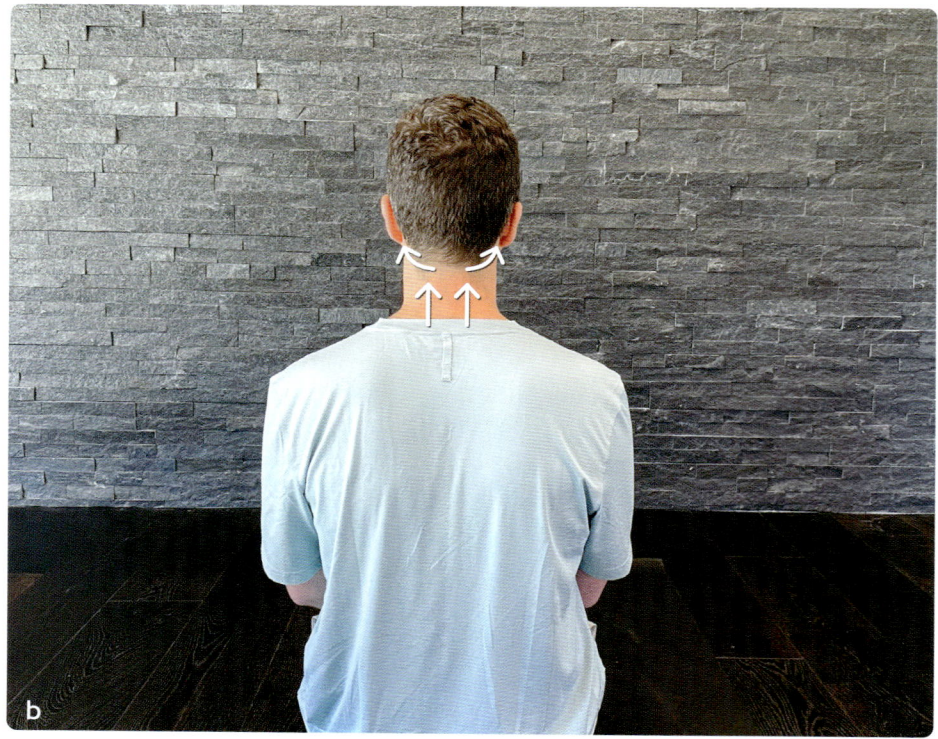

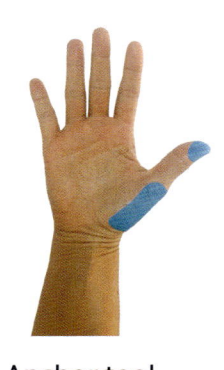

Anchor tool

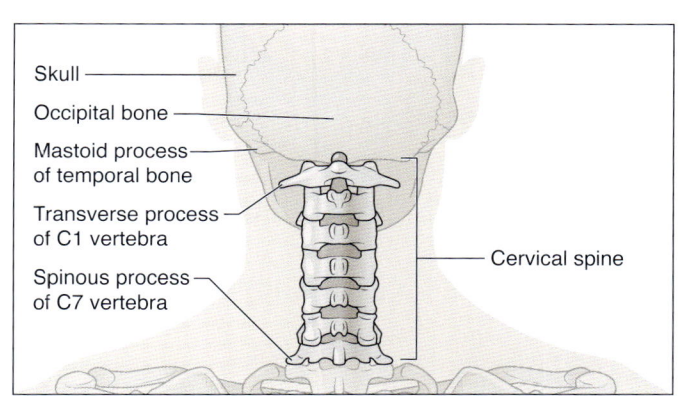

Skull
Occipital bone
Mastoid process of temporal bone
Transverse process of C1 vertebra
Spinous process of C7 vertebra

Cervical spine

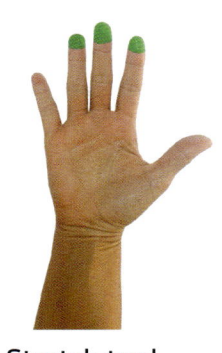

Stretch tool

Skull
Rectus capitis posterior minor
Mastoid process of temporal bone
Rectus capitis posterior major
Transverse process of C1 vertebra
Obliquus capitis inferior
Longissimus capitis
Trapezius (cut) :
Descending fibers
Transverse fibers
Ascending fibers

Semispinalis capitis
Sternocleidomastoid
Splenius capitis
Spinous process of C7 vertebra
Splenius cervicis
Levator scapulae
First rib
Shoulder girdle:
Clavicle
Scapula
Acromioclavicular joint
Glenohumeral joint
Humeral head
Humerus
Rhomboid minor
Rhomboid major

■ Anchor placement
■ Stretch placement

Corpse Pose: Neck Traction

Purpose

Corpse pose, or savasana, is intended to cultivate relaxation and integration of the practice. However, many students struggle to remain present in this pose because their minds wander and drift off. An assist can help the student remain grounded and easeful in the pose. Working with the neck can be extremely relaxing, amplifying the grounding and presence students cultivate in this pose. This assist also stretches the tissues at the back of the neck.

Stance

Easy Seat
Alternative: Low Squat

Sit close enough to your student that when you lean forward to place your elbows on your legs, your fingertips can touch the tops of your student's shoulders. Your elbows remain on your legs throughout the assist.

Anchor Tool: Provided by the Student

The student's head and shoulders generally act as the anchors. If necessary, add additional anchoring by steadying the student's head with the base of your thumb or thumb tips. The head remains still on the mat throughout the assist.

Anchor Placement: Behind the Ears

If you are using both thumbs to steady the student's head, gently allow them to remain at the base of the skull (occiput) or the bony protrusion behind the ears (mastoid process of the temporal bone). You can place your thumbs here before you begin the spinal traction or use them to steady the student's head if it starts to move during the assist.

Stretch Tool: Fingertips, Generally Only Ring, Middle, and Index Fingers

Turn your palms upward and curl your fingers as if holding a bowl. You will use the soft finger pads of your index, middle, and ring fingers to provide the stretch.

Stretch Placement: Base of Cervical Spine, C7

Find vertebra C7 on yourself before attempting this assist. Along your spine, where the shoulders meet the neck, there is a vertebra that is larger than the others. This is C7 and the starting place for this assist.

Find the C7 spinous process. Using the pads of your index, middle, and ring fingers, place your fingers on the right and left sides of the spine, starting at this large C7 vertebra. Your finger pads will sink into soft tissue on either side of C7. To hook into the tissue, press your fingers slowly toward the ceiling and into your student's tissue. The pressure is just enough to sink into the tissue without causing the student's neck and head to move or lift.

Follow the Lines

You are following the lines of your student's skeleton, drawing a *T* shape along the length of the cervical spine and then along the base of the skull (occipital bone).

Starting around C7, slowly slide your finger pads up the length of the neck on either side of the spine. Your fingers will eventually reach the hairline and base of the skull (occipital bone).

When you feel the ledge of the occipital bone or the soft depression where the spine meets the skull, you will change direction with your fingers. If you were to trace a line along the back of your student's neck and head, it would look like your two hands drew a *T* up the spine and out to the right and left at the base of the skull.

Once your fingers have reached the base of the skull or the inferior edge of the occiput, turn them slightly inward. When you started, your wrists and fingers pointed toward the student's toes. Now, as you turn to draw the upper portion of the *T*, angle your hands inward so your fingers face each other, allowing you to follow the base of the skull from the center outward to the left and right.

Once you have turned your fingers, instead of sliding along the base of the skull, palpate along the base of the skull to avoid massaging or pulling the student's hair. With both hands moving laterally (to the left and right), press the soft tissue at the inferior ridge of the occiput. Palpate a few times until you reach the mastoid process, the bony protrusion behind the ears.

Myofascial Region

The myofascia compressed and stretched in this assist includes the cervical erector spinae (spinalis, longissimus, iliocostalis), splenius capitis, descending trapezius, and suboccipital muscles.

General Precautions

The intention isn't to pull the neck but to lengthen the soft tissues that hug the sides of the spine. Avoid lifting or moving the head or trying to pull the neck and head toward you.

Common Misalignments

There are no common misalignments with this pose. However, you should generally avoid offering neck work to someone with cervical spine injuries or pain. Also, if a student has their head propped up on anything more than a flat blanket, don't offer this assist.

Troubleshooting

Each student's neck is unique. You may find that some feel as through they have very little muscle tissue, whereas others have lots, and students may have more or less pliable skin on the neck.

If someone has a lot of muscular tissue, the assist will require a little more "sinking in." If they have less, you won't need to sink in as much. If they have a lot of loose skin, go even slower when you provide traction to the neck. If you do not rush, the tissue will lengthen on its own.

You want the head and neck to remain neutral. This means you are not picking the student's head up off the floor. The chin must not sink toward the throat and chest but remain in neutral to indicate that the cervical spine is also in neutral.

PUTTING IT ALL TOGETHER

- Find an easy seat behind your student.
- Be fully in your student's space, only a few inches away, so that you do not feel like you must reach to find the base of their neck.
- Lean forward and allow your elbows to rest on your legs. With your forearms and fingers extended towards the student, you should just be able to touch the tops of their shoulders.
- With your index, middle, and ring fingers, find either side of C7 at the base of your student's neck.
- Place your thumbs on the bony protrusion behind their ears to rest on the mastoid process. With your thumbs, lightly steady the head in place.
- Curl your fingers into the tissues on either side of the spine at the C7 vertebra and begin to draw your fingers toward you to provide traction to the length of the neck or cervical spine.
- Slowly provide traction to either side of the spine until you feel an indentation of soft tissue just inferior to the bony ridge at the base of the skull. Pause momentarily here.
- Rotate your fingers and shift the directional pressure from upward (superior) to outward (lateral). With a palpating motion, so as not to pull the student's hair, palpate a few times, moving along the soft tissue directly inferior to the occiput. Your fingers will stop around the mastoid processes behind the ears.
- Pause and press near the mastoid process to complete the lines of the *T* that you traced up the spine and out toward the ears.
- To complete the assist, gently release the fingers first and thumbs last to avoid disturbing the head as much as possible.

Deer Pose: Reverse Shoulder Press

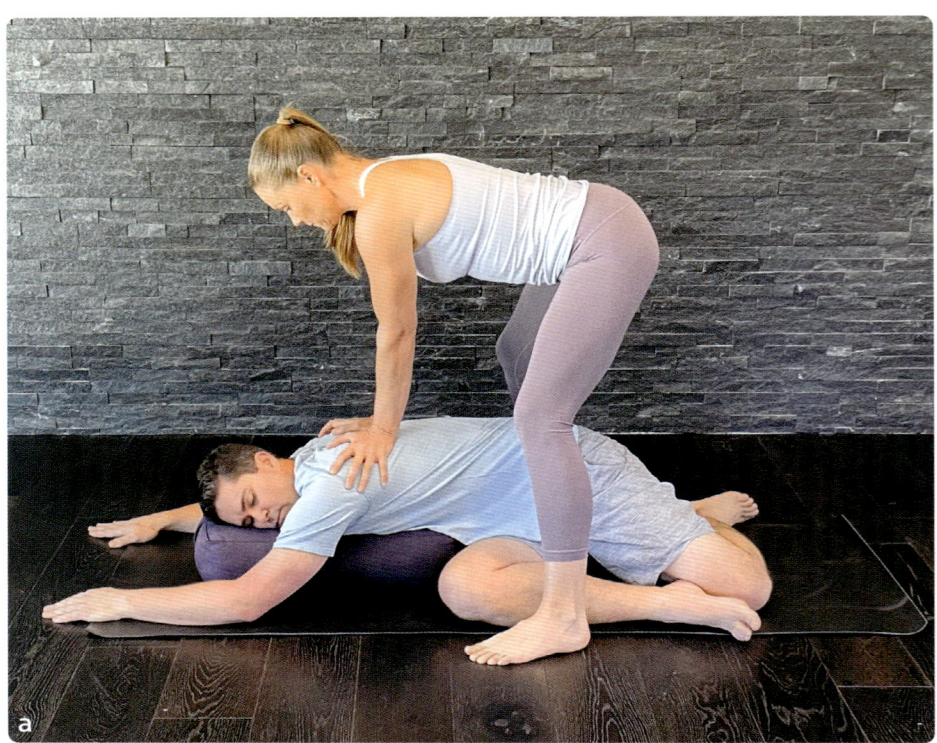

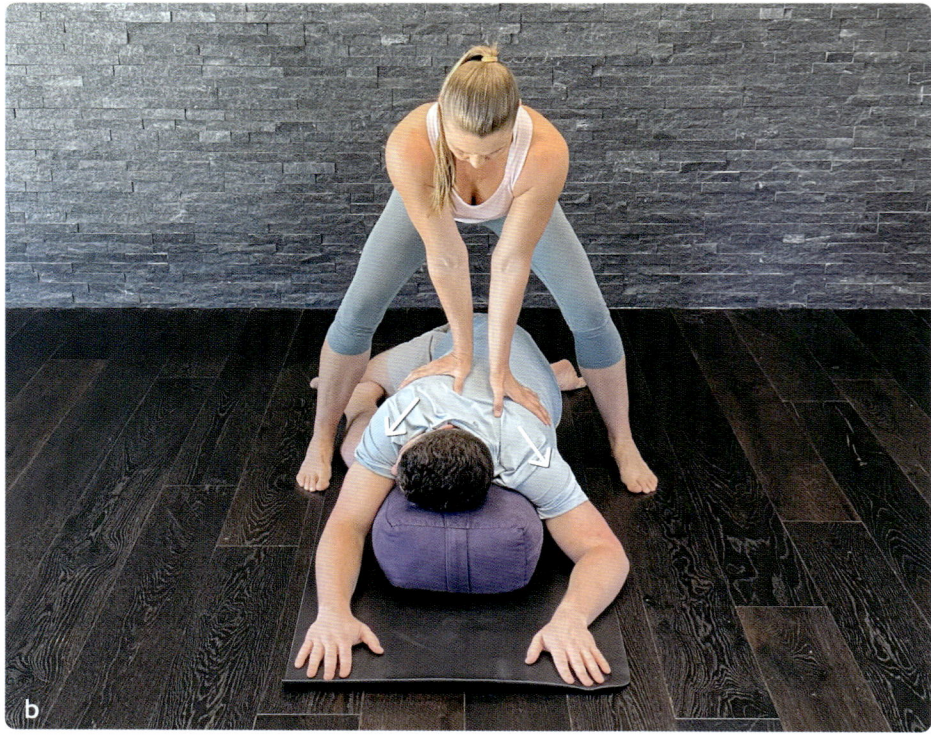

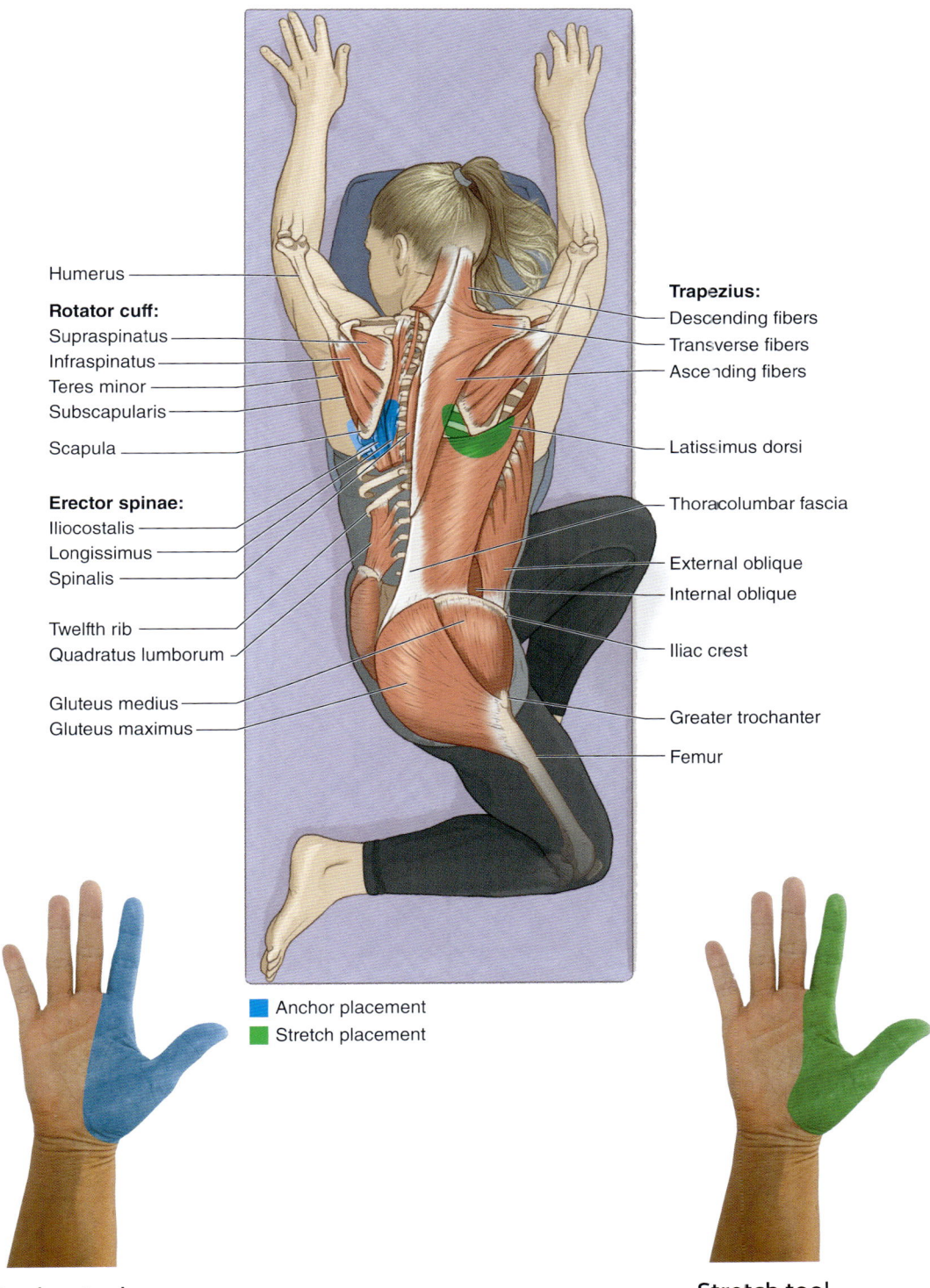

Humerus

Rotator cuff:
Supraspinatus
Infraspinatus
Teres minor
Subscapularis

Scapula

Erector spinae:
Iliocostalis
Longissimus
Spinalis

Twelfth rib
Quadratus lumborum

Gluteus medius
Gluteus maximus

Trapezius:
Descending fibers
Transverse fibers
Ascending fibers

Latissimus dorsi

Thoracolumbar fascia

External oblique
Internal oblique

Iliac crest

Greater trochanter

Femur

■ Anchor placement
■ Stretch placement

Anchor tool

Stretch tool

STUDENT ALIGNMENT

Mrigasana: Deer Pose

The legs are either scissored or stacked one on top of the other.

The torso is fully supported by a bolster running parallel to the student's spine.

Both shoulders are squared toward the bolster.

The arms extend toward the top of the mat; the elbows are ahead of the shoulders.

The head is rotated either toward or away from the knees, based on the student's comfort.

Purpose

Deer pose on a bolster emphasizes protraction, creating opening in the upper back. A reverse shoulder press accentuates the lines of stretch between the scapulae (shoulder blades). The assist also offers a heightened sense of the grounding felt in this restorative pose.

Stance

High Squat

Step over your student and roughly align your heels with your student's midthighs, adjusting this based on your height. When you bend your knees and send your hips back, your shoulders should be directly over your student's shoulders. Keep your arms straight throughout the assist.

Anchor Tool: Thenar Eminence (Base of Thumb)

Offer this assist with alternating pressure from side to side. As one hand applies pressure, the opposite hand backs off the pressure but remains in place to stabilize the student. The stabilization is the anchor and counterbalance to the pressure applied by the stretch hand. With this alternating pressure, the anchor and stretch hands alternate in this assist.

Anchor Placement

Place the anchor on the soft tissue along the medial border and inferior angle of the scapulae. See Stretch Placement.

Stretch Tool: Thenar Eminence (Base of Thumb)

Turn your palms downward and angle your hands outward so that your thumbs point toward the student's head and your fingers point out to the sides. Your thumbs will point toward 12 o'clock, and your fingers will point toward 3 o'clock and 9 o'clock. You will mostly use the base of your thumb to offer the stretch, but the whole hand can rest on the student's back. The shape of your tool, or hand, mimics the shape of the student's scapula.

Stretch Placement: Transverse Ascending Fibers of Trapezius, Latissimus Dorsi; Soft Tissue Bordering Medial Border and Inferior Angle of the Scapulae

Look for the medial borders and inferior angles of the scapulae. These are the inner edges and bottom tips of the shoulder blades, respectively. Your thumbs will run along the medial border of the scapula, with your index finger running along the inferior angle and lateral border. The space between the index finger and thumb curves along the inferior angle. Using the base of your thumb, gently press in toward the rib cage to hook into the myofascia bordering the bony landmarks of the scapulae.

Follow the Lines

The assist aims to broaden the upper back. The lines of stretch follow the transverse (middle) and ascending (lower) fibers of the trapezius muscle. The trapezius looks a lot like a diamond or kite. You can imagine this shape running from the base of the skull, spreading outward across the shoulders, spanning between the shoulder blades, and down to the lower thoracic spine. By applying directional pressure to the medial shoulder blades outward with a broadening intention, you target the middle and lower fibers of this muscle. Alternate pressure with each hand at a diagonal angled toward the head of each shoulder or each respective elbow.

For the student to have suitable alignment for an assist, their arms need to be reaching forward but relaxed. Although they do not feel the assist in their arms, the lines continue from the scapula of the shoulder out through the fingertips.

Alternate the pressure of the assist from side to side. When alternating pressure, keep both hands on the student. Do not lift one hand and press with the other; keep both hands on the student until you have completed the assist. The hand applying pressure applies the stretch. The opposite hand provides a counterbalance and the anchor. With enough stabilizing pressure in the anchor, while applying the directional pressure of the stretch, you will feel the tissue between the two points become taut and stretch. When alternating pressure from side to side, be mindful to have a slow rhythm to your palpation.

Myofascial Region

This assist involves myofascia in the thoracic region or upper and middle back, specifically the transverse fibers and ascending fibers of the trapezius. The latissimus dorsi muscle will also receive some compression and stretch.

General Precautions

This is generally a safe assist to offer any student. However, if a student has a shoulder or neck injury, it's always best to avoid offering shoulder assists.

This assist may not be appropriate in trauma-informed yoga settings.

Common Misalignments

If a student cannot rotate fully and place their chest on the bolster, do not offer this assist. You may need to offer the student a block beneath their bolster for more elevation and support in this spinal twist. A student who cannot twist completely will usually look as though they are lying sideways with one shoulder on their bolster. This student needs an adjustment in their props rather than a Rubber Band Method® assist.

Troubleshooting

Many students will pull their elbows toward their sides in this shape, as if hugging the bolster. If you apply pressure near the shoulder blade, this will press the student's elbow into the floor. This is uncomfortable for the student and can cause the assist to move into their neck. Consider gently moving the student's arms and elbow forward a bit, or use cuing to invite them to reach their arms farther forward and then relax their arms.

The range of motion in scapulae can vary considerably from student to student. Be sure to look for the bony landmarks of the scapula to help you identify the handhold. The scapulae are not always located close to the spine; in flexible students, they are often upwardly rotated a great deal away from the spine.

PUTTING IT ALL TOGETHER

- Step over your student and find a high-squat stance with your heels roughly aligned with the student's midthighs.

- Bend your knees, keeping your back straight, and lean forward to align your shoulders over your student's shoulders.

- Visually find your student's scapulae (shoulder blades) and note the inner (medial) border of each. Look for the bony ridge closest to the spine. This is where your thumb will go.

- Turn your palms down and angle your hands so that your thumbs point toward the student's head and your fingers point out to the sides, or toward the student's shoulders. Place the base of your thumb just inside each scapula. Your thumbs will run parallel with the medial border of the scapulae, and your index finger and palm will wrap along the inferior angle and lateral border of the scapulae.

- Keep your arms straight as you apply pressure to the student's rib cage with the base of your thumb. This allows you to hook into their tissue and establish a good handhold.

- Alternate pressure between hands, but do not remove your hands. Press slightly into the ribs and then out toward the shoulder head. Apply directional pressure toward the student or down and then out toward the student's shoulders or elbows. Use your legs by shifting your weight into either foot as you alternate pressure from side to side.

- It should feel as though the pressure you are applying is spreading the upper back wider. Stop when you feel any resistance from the myofascia or the shoulder blades themselves.

- Just before ending the assist, apply pressure with both hands simultaneously while reducing the overall pressure. Exit the assist slowly, guiding the student's tissues back to their natural resting position before removing both hands simultaneously.

REFERENCES

Chapter 1

1. Packheiser J, Hartmann H, Fredriksen K, et al. A systematic review and multivariate meta-analysis of the physical and mental health benefits of touch interventions. *Nat Hum Behav.* 2024;8:1088-1107. https://doi.org/10.1038/s41562-024-01841-8.

Chapter 2

1. *American Heritage Dictionary of the English Language.* 5th ed. Boston: Houghton Mifflin Harcourt; 2016. www.thefreedictionary.com/adjust.

2. *American Heritage Dictionary of the English Language.* 5th ed. Boston: Houghton Mifflin Harcourt; 2016. www.thefreedictionary.com/assist.

Chapter 4

1. Leemis RW, Friar N, Khatiwada S, et al. *The National Intimate Partner and Sexual Violence Survey: 2016/2017 Report on Intimate Partner Violence.* Atlanta, GA: Centers for Disease Control and Prevention, National Center for Injury Prevention and Control; 2022.

2. Kearl, Holly. *The Facts Behind the #MeToo Movement: A National Study on Sexual Harassment and Assault.* Reston, VA: Stop Street Harassment; 2018.

3. Rape, Abuse & Incest National Network (RAINN). 2023. "*Children and Teens: Statistics on Sexual Violence.*" Accessed February 25, 2025. https://rainn.org/statistics/children-and-teens.

4. World Health Organization. *Violence Against Women Prevalence Estimates, 2018.* Geneva, Switzerland: WHO; 2021.

5. UNICEF. 2024. "*Over 370 Million Girls and Women Globally Subjected to Rape or Sexual Assault as Children.*" Published October 10, 2024. Accessed March 19, 2025. https://www.unicef.org/press-releases/over-370-million-girls-and-women-globally-subjected-rape-or-sexual-assault-children. Kessler, Ronald C., Sergio Aguilar-Gaxiola, Jordi Alonso, Corina Benjet, Evelyn J. Bromet, Graça Cardoso, Louisa Degenhardt, Giovanni de Girolamo, Rumyana V. Dinolova, Finola Ferry, Silvia Florescu, Oye Gureje, Josep Maria Haro, Yueqin Huang, Elie G. Karam, Norito Kawakami, Sing Lee, Jean-Pierre Lepine, Daphna Levinson, Fernando Navarro-Mateu, Beth-Ellen Pennell, Marina Piazza, José Posada-Villa, Kate M. Scott, Dan J. Stein, Maria Carmen Viana, and Karestan C. Koenen. 2017. "Trauma and PTSD in the WHO World Mental Health Surveys." *European Journal of Psychotraumatology* 8 (sup5): 1353383. https://doi.org/10.1080/20008198.2017.1353383.

Chapter 5

1. Packheiser J, Hartmann H, Fredriksen K, et al. A systematic review and multivariate meta-analysis of the physical and mental health benefits of touch interventions. *Nat Hum Behav.* 2024;8:1088-1107. https://doi.org/10.1038/s41562-024-01841-8.

2. Van der Kolk B. *The Body Keeps the Score.* New York: Penguin Books; 2015, pp. 315-317.

ABOUT THE AUTHOR

Kiara Armstrong, **E-RYT 500, CMT, YACEP,** first started practicing yoga in 2002. It played a central role in her personal journey to overcome mental and physical illness. In 2010, she began her first 200-hour yoga teacher training and started teaching in 2011. Five years later, she began leading 200-hour yoga teacher trainings and has since taught continuing education programs, including 300-hour yoga teacher trainings. She has a deep reverence for the human body, having spent time working independently with a cadaver and sharing her knowledge as an anatomy instructor in both yoga and massage schools. In addition to being an E-RYT 500 registered teacher with Yoga Alliance, she is a certified massage therapist. Her experience working with clients in a medical setting has given her a more intimate understanding of the body—one that extends beyond what is visible in a yoga classroom.

Kiara's love for hands-on assists began early in her yoga practice when she was introduced to them in structured, traditional settings. Over the years, she encountered a wide range of assisting styles—some that felt profoundly helpful and others that left her questioning their safety and effectiveness. At times, she experienced strains and injuries from well-intentioned but imprecise touch interventions, which led her to explore the mechanics of assisting more deeply. As an employee of *Yoga Journal* magazine, she was exposed to a variety of teachers who employed different approaches to hands-on techniques, further reinforcing the need for a system that was clear, teachable, and adaptable to different body types and classroom environments.

Her search for a structured approach led her to formal Thai massage training, which provided valuable insight but ultimately did not translate seamlessly to a yoga setting. She continued experimenting, refining her understanding through thousands of hours of teaching and hands-on experience. Slowly, through practice, observation, and adaptation, the Rubber Band Method® was born. This method makes a clear distinction between assisting and adjusting, recognizing that while both have a place in yoga instruction, they are not interchangeable. Kiara developed a systematic approach that prioritizes sustainable body mechanics for the teacher, purposeful and intuitive touch for the student, and the ability to read tissues through tactile awareness.

Through years of trial, refinement, and student feedback, Rubber Band Method® evolved into a structured, accessible system that any yoga instructor can learn and apply with confidence. Designed to prioritize both student safety and teacher sustainability, it provides a clear framework for offering hands-on support that is intuitive, effective, and respectful of each individual's body. Kiara continues to refine and share this approach with the goal of making safe, skillful assisting an integral part of modern yoga education—one that can stand on its own and be passed on for generations to come.

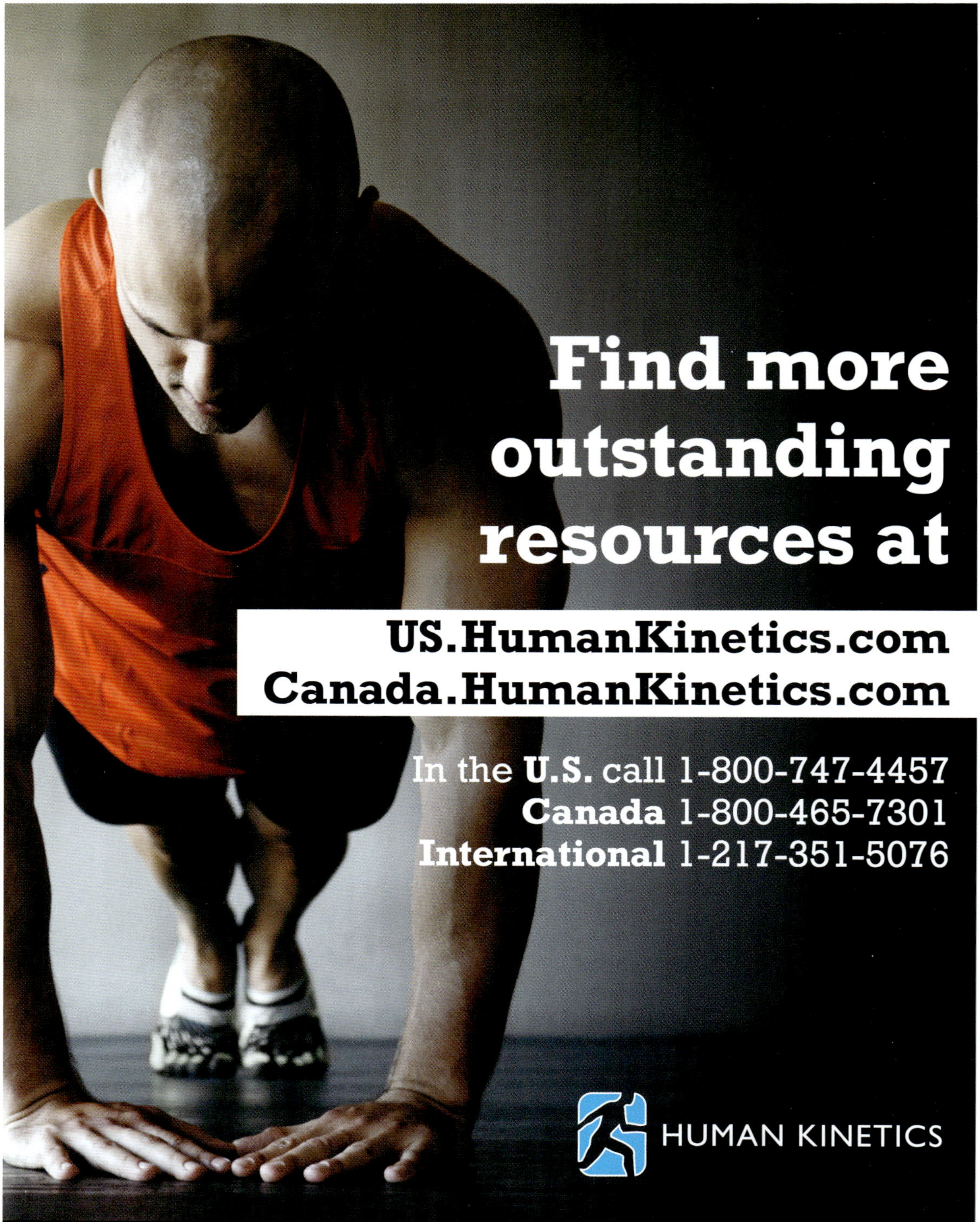